THE FAMILY NUTRITION WORKBOOK

The type and quality of the food you eat is of direct relevance to your health, and it is something that you can take immediate action to improve. By reading this book you will not only get a solid foundation in nutrition, but you will also get healthier and more alert in the process. Includes a section on working out your ideal supplement programme.

THE
FAMILY NUTRITION
WORKBOOK

All the facts about food you need to know
for a healthy family

by

Patrick Holford B.Sc.

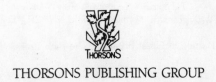
THORSONS PUBLISHING GROUP

First published 1988

British Library Cataloguing in Publication Data

Holford, Patrick
The nutrition workbook
1. Nutrition   2. Health
I. Title
613.2   RA784

ISBN 0-7225-1466-2

*Published by Thorsons Publishers Limited,
Wellingborough, Northamptonshire, NN8 2RQ, England*

Printed in Great Britain at The Bath Press, Avon

3 5 7 9 10 8 6 4

Contents

Acknowledgements

This book could not have been written without the help and support of my friends and colleagues. I would particularly like to thank Tony Searby for his help in writing Chapters 2.3 and 3.8; David Stevens and Janet Anders for their help in writing Chapter 1.2; Liz, my wife, and Ebury Press for allowing me to use adapted extracts from *The Metabolic Diet* and *The Better Pregnancy Diet*; Collins for allowing me to adapt a chapter on choosing your vitamin needs from *Vitamin Vitality*; and most of all Chris Scarfe and Jill Stokes for running the Institute in my absence. I would also like to thank Thorsons for their support and patience.

A special thank-you goes to Chris Quayle for his excellent diagrams and illustrations.

Figure 1.2.6 is reproduced from *The Metabolic Diet* by kind permission of Ebury press, and figures 1.2.7 and 3.8.1 are reproduced from *Vitamin Vitality* by kind permission of Collins.

PART ONE

— Introduction To Nutrition —

CHAPTER 1.1

How healthy do you want to be?

Everyone has a different idea of what health is and how healthy they'd like to be. Although we use the word almost every day it isn't easy to define. It's a lot easier to define what health isn't than say what it is. It isn't aches and pains, it isn't headaches, it isn't feeling tired half way through the day and it certainly isn't feeling ill. If you were to make a list of all the qualities that went with being healthy you'd probably include some of those listed below:

lack of obvious illness
sense of well-being
feeling full of energy
feeling calm and unstressed
having no physical discomfort.

One of my patients described being healthy as being 'blissfully oblivious of myself all day long!' But health is also a matter of expectation. Many people expect to have to wear glasses by the age of fifty, or to have a few joint aches and pains. Until recently women expected to experience some sort of pre-menstrual tension. To these people, you can still be healthy and suffer from these 'normal', 'expected' health problems.

Other people appear relatively free from the symptoms we associate with ill-health, but then suffer a heart attack or are diagnosed as having cancer quite out of the blue. Could it be that these people were really unhealthy but just didn't know about it? Or did the disease really strike out of the blue, and if so, why? All the evidence points

to the former explanation. Diseases like cancer and heart disease take years to develop. Despite being symptom free these unfortunate people were unconsciously fighting a losing battle and one day their bodies ran out of reserves.

At the other end of the scale we have to ask what is the ultimate we can experience in the way of health. I have had the opportunity to study extremely healthy people. Top athletes, top intellects and people with alert minds and bodies late into life. From these studies it is clear that the experiences that many people accept as normal are far from right. From these healthy people we can get a taste of what is possible and indeed probable if one's lifestyle is a healthy one. It may surprise you to know that some gerontologists believe that our maximum achievable lifespan is certainly more than 110. Memory and mental function should not decline drastically with age; blood-pressure and pulse should not go up substantially with age; in women, the menopause should not occur before age fifty-five and even so, should not produce unpleasant associated symptoms; pre-menstrual symptoms should also be scarcely noticeable; a pregnant woman should not feel sick during pregnancy. Yet so rare is it for us to know someone with this level of health our tendency is to dismiss these scientific facts as wishful thinking.

By examining what health is it becomes clear the answer is not that straightforward. At least the following key factors would need to be met in order to qualify as super-healthy.

Health is . . . being symptom free
having physical reserves to fight off disease
a real sense of well-being
reaching for one's maximum potential for mental and physical performance.

How to become healthy

Having defined what health is, how do you become healthy? You might start by making a list of all the different factors that affect your health and how you feel. Your list will probably include some of the following:

Diet
Exercise
Job satisfaction
Addictions (i.e. smoking, coffee)
Pollution and environment
Amount of stress
Inherited weaknesses
Exposure to infections
Alcohol consumption
Relationships
Relaxation and leisure time
Sunshine
Temperature
Sense of purpose, direction

Some of these relate to physical things: sunshine, diet, exercise, pollution. Others are psychological: relaxation, job satisfaction, relationships. It soon becomes clear on the physical side that everything you eat, breathe, drink and are exposed to could have a bearing on your health. In the broadest sense, this is what optimum nutrition is all about. Studying what our bodies need, and don't need, to stay in top form.

But it is impossible to totally separate the physical and the psychological. After all, every thought process or emotion changes our body chemistry, and every ingestion of food can, in turn, affect our mood or thinking processes. Alcohol releases inhibition and can be a depressant. Coffee improves reaction time. Foods high in the amino acid tryptophan can make you feel drowsy. Conversely, what we eat depends to a large extent on how we feel psychologically. Many people crave food when they are bored or depressed. We serve food to make guests welcome, and as an expression of thanks.

So there's a lot more to eating than feeling hungry and a lot more to health than just eating the right foods. But having said that, good nutrition is a fundamental element of a healthy lifestyle and an important starting point, and has been recognized as such for at least two thousand years. 'Let food be your medicine and medicine your food', said Hippocrates in 460 BC.

Assess your own health

What is ideal for one person isn't necessarily ideal for everybody. So we've devised a questionnaire called the Nutrition Programme Questionnaire which will help you to find out how healthy you are and how healthy you could be, and it will provide the impetus for the achievement of optimum nutrition.

But what is optimum nutrition? This whole book is about that question. There must be a starting point. That starting point is to examine how we, as a species, have evolved to need nutrients. With this information it becomes possible to alter our nutrition to conform as closely as possible to our design. In the next chapter we examine the nature of the human organism and our origins, which help to define more exactly what optimum nutrition is.

Nutrition Programme Questionnaire

Health Profile

Make a list of all the health problems you would like to clear up, and indicate how long you have had these problems: e.g. headaches, 5 years.

Health problem   Duration

1. _____   _____

2. _____   _____

3. _____   _____

4. _____   _____

5. _____   _____

6. _____   _____

7. _____   _____

8. _____   _____

9. _____   _____

10. _____   _____

What medications (drugs) do you take for these? State daily dosage.
_____

Under what circumstances do these problems improve?
_____

Under what circumstances do they get worse?
_____

What other illnesses have you had in the past ten years?
_____

What operations have you had? _____

What is your normal blood pressure? _____
(don't worry if you don't know)

What is your resting pulse rate per minute?_____
(YOU SHOULD BE SITTING DOWN, RELAXED AND CALM WHEN YOU TAKE YOUR PULSE.
YOUR PULSE CAN BE FOUND INSIDE THE BONY PROTUBERANCE ON THE THUMB SIDE
OF YOUR WRIST. COUNT THE NUMBER OF BEATS IN 60 SECONDS.)

Vitamin and Mineral Profile

Each question in this section starts with a list of symptoms associated with nutritional deficiency. Please underline the conditions you often suffer from. Some symptoms are repeated. Please underline them in all cases.

Mouth ulcers
Poor night vision
Acne
Frequent colds or infections
Dry flaky skin
Dandruff
Thrush or cystitis
Diarrhoea

Rheumatism or arthritis
Backache
Tooth decay
Hair loss
Excessive sweating
Muscle cramps, tremors or spasms
Joint pain or stiffness
Lack of energy

Lack of sex drive
Exhaustion after light exercise
Easy bruising
Slow wound healing
Varicose veins
Loss of muscle tone
Infertility

Frequent colds
Lack of energy
Frequent infections
Bleeding or tender gums
Easy bruising
Nose bleeds
Slow wound healing
Red pimples on skin

Poor concentration
Irritability
Depression
Anxiety or tension
Poor skin condition
Lack of energy
Headaches

Tender muscles
Eye pains
Irritability
Poor concentration
'Prickly' legs
Poor memory
Stomach pains
Constipation
Tingling hands
Rapid heart beat

Bloodshot, burning or gritty eyes
Sensitivity to bright lights
Sore tongue
Cataracts
Dull or oily hair
Eczema or dermatitis
Split nails
Cracked lips

Lack of energy
Diarrhoea
Insomnia
Headaches or migraines
Poor memory
Anxiety or tension
Depression
Irritability
Bleeding or tender gums
Acne

Muscle tremors, cramps or spasms
Apathy
Poor concentration
Burning feet or tender heels
Nausea or vomiting
Lack of energy
Exhaustion after light exercise
Anxiety or tension
Teeth grinding

Infrequent dream recall
Water retention
Tingling hands
Depression or nervousness
Irritability
Muscle tremors, cramps or spasms
Lack of energy

Poor hair condition
Eczema or dermatitis
Mouth over-sensitive to hot or cold
Irritability
Anxiety or tension
Lack of energy
Constipation
Tender or sore muscles
Pale skin

Eczema
Cracked lips
Prematurely greying hair
Anxiety or tension
Poor memory
Lack of energy
Depression
Poor appetite
Stomach pains
Poor memory
Hand or head tremor
Depression
Frequent colds

Poor hair condition
Prematurely greying hair
Frequent sunburn
Irritability
Stomach pains

Dermatitis or dry skin
Poor hair condition
Prematurely greying hair
Tender or sore muscles
Poor appetite or nausea

Muscle cramps, tremors or spasms
Insomnia or nervousness
Joint pain or arthritis
Tooth decay
High blood pressure

Pale skin
Sore tongue
Fatigue or listlessness
Loss of appetite or nausea
Heavy periods or blood loss

Decline in sense of taste or smell
White marks on more than two finger nails
Frequent infections
Stretch marks
Acne or greasy skin

Muscle twitches
Childhood 'growing pains'
Dizziness or poor sense of balance
Fits or convulsions
Sore knees

Family history of cancer
Signs of premature aging
Cataracts
High blood pessure

Excessive or cold sweats
Dizziness or irritability after six hours without food
Need for frequent meals
Cold hands

Need for excessive sleep or drowsiness during the day

Hereditary Profile

Do you have any children? If so, state age and sex.

How many brothers or sisters do you have? State age and sex.

Are there any particular illnesses that they suffer from?

What illnesses is/was your father prone to?

What illnesses is/was your mother prone to?

Additional Questions for Women Only

_____Are you pregnant? If so how many weeks?

_____Are you trying to become pregnant? If so, how long have you been trying?

_____Have you ever had a miscarriage?

_____Do you have an IUD fitted, or use the birth control pill? State which. _____

_____Are your periods regular?

_____Are you post-menopausal?

Do you suffer from any of the following before at least three out of five periods? Please underline.

Bloatedness, tiredness, irritability, depression, breast tenderness, headaches.

Stress Profile (For Men and Women)

_____Do you feel guilty when relaxing?

_____Do you have a persistent need for recognition and achievement?

_____Are you unclear about your goals in life?

_____Are you especially competitive?

_____Do you work harder than most people?

_____Do you easily become angry?

_____Are you always in a hurry?

_____Do you often do two or three tasks simultaneously?

_____Do you get impatient if people hold you up?

_____Do you find it especially difficult to openly admit failure or defeat?

Cardiovascular Profile

_____Is your blood pressure above 140/90?

_____Is your pulse after 15 minute's rest above 75?

_____Are you more than 14lbs over your ideal weight?

_____Do you smoke more than five cigarettes a day?

_____Do you do less than two hours (one hour if you're over 50) of vigorous exercise a week?

_____Do you eat more than one tablespoon of sugar each day?

_____Is your lifestyle very stressful?

_____Is there a history of heart disease in your family?

_____Do you eat meat, not fish, more than five times a week?

_____Do you ever get palpitations or irregular heart beats?

Exercise Profile

_____Do you take exercise that noticeably raises your heart beat for 20 minutes more than three times a week?

_____Does your job involve lots of walking, lifting or any other vigorous activity?

_____Do you regularly play a sport? (football, squash, etc.)

_____Do you have any physically tiring hobbies?

_____Are you in serious training for an athletic event?

_____Do you consider yourself fit?

Glucose Tolerance Profile

_____Do you sweat a lot during the night or day?

_____Do you experience dizziness or irritability if you go six hours without eating?

_____Do you regularly feel drowsy or sleepy in the day?

_____Do you always need a coffee, tea or something sweet to get you going in the morning?

_____Do you frequently get headaches?

_____Do you get cold hands?

_____Are you frequently anxious, fearful or depressed?

_____Do you need frequent meals or snacks?

_____Are you often thirsty?

_____Do you have difficulty digesting fatty foods?

Histamine Profile

Underline the following that apply to you:

Sleep more than eight hours	*Sleep less than seven hours*
Little sex drive	*Strong sex drive*
Much body hair	*Little body hair*
Infrequent colds	*Family history of allergies*
Sluggish metabolism	
Slow to wake up	*Fast metabolism*

Short toes and fingers	*'Morning' person*
Suspicious by nature	*Long toes and fingers*
Fat or 'well covered'	*Tends towards depression*
Can tolerate pain	*Don't put on weight*
	Poor tolerance to pain

Allergy Profile

Do you suffer from any of the following? Please underline.

Rhinitis, hay fever, post-nasal drip, eczema, dermatitis, asthma, migraine, irritable bowel syndrome, frequent bloatedness, facial puffiness.

Do you have any allergies? If so to what?
_____

State type of reaction._____

How have they been tested?_____

Are there any other substances you react to?
_____

What food or drinks would you find hard to give up? _____

Pollution Risk Profile

_____Do you live in a city or by a busy road?

_____Do you smoke more than five cigarettes a day?

_____Do you spend more than two hours a week in heavy traffic?

_____Do you exercise by busy roads?

_____Do you live in a new (less than one year) or old (pre-1940) house?

_____Do you live in a soft water area?

_____Do you drink more than one alcoholic drink a day?

_____Do you occasionally use indigestion tablets?

_____Do you have aluminium or copper pots and pans?

_____Do you have more than five amalgam (silver) fillings?

Please tick the questions to which you would answer 'yes' or fill in the number of times you eat the food referred to in the question.

_____ 1. Do you go out of your way to avoid foods containing additives?

_____ 2. Do you avoid foods which contain sugar?

_____ 3. How many teaspoons of sugar do you add to food/drinks each day?

_____ 4. Do you use salt in your cooking?

_____ 5. Do you add salt to your food?

_____ 6. How many cups of coffee do you drink each day?

_____ 7. How many cups of tea do you drink each day?

_____ 8. How many times a week do you have meals containing fried food?

_____ 9. How many packets of 'instant' or fast foods do you eat each week?

_____ 10. How many times a week do you eat chocolate or confectionary?

_____ 11. What percentage of your diet is raw fruit and raw vegetables?

_____ 12. Do you wash fresh fruit and vegetables before eating them?

_____ 13. Do you normally eat refined rice or flour?

_____ 14. How many cans of food do you eat per week?

_____ 15. How many slices of bread do you eat per week?

_____ 16. How many pints of milk do you drink in a week?

_____ 17. How many times a week do you eat red meat? (beef, pork, lamb or game)

_____ 18. How many times a week do you eat white meat? (poultry, fish)

_____ 19. What is your usual alcoholic drink?

_____ 20. How many glasses do you drink a week?

_____ 21. How many times a week do you eat natural yogurt?

_____ 22. Do you use a water filter or drink bottled water instead of tap water?

Diet Profile

Write down all the foods and drinks consumed over the next three days, starting today. Please add as much information as possible including quantities eaten, brand names, and whether the food is fresh or packaged, refined or natural.

Day 1

BREAKFAST

What Nutritional Supplements do you take daily on a regular basis?

LUNCH

Are these three days representative of your usual eating habits? If not, what is a more usual day?

DINNER

BREAKFAST

SNACKS/DRINKS

LUNCH

DINNER

Day 2
BREAKFAST   SNACKS/DRINKS

LUNCH

DINNER

SNACKS/DRINKS

Day 3
BREAKFAST

LUNCH

DINNER

SNACKS/DRINKS

CHAPTER 1.2

Understanding optimum nutrition

What are you made of?

Everything we see (and everything we don't) is made up of tiny particles called atoms. The simplest of these is hydrogen, which is made up of two very small particles called a proton and an electron. (More complex atoms have more electrons and protons, as well as other large particles called neutrons.) As more particles are added to the atom, the way in which it behaves and reacts with other atoms around it changes. These different sized atoms are called elements, and we know of over 100 different atoms and elements all of which have different characteristics. The most important ones, as far as life is concerned, are oxygen, carbon, hydrogen and nitrogen.

The basic building blocks of life are composed of combinations of these four important atoms.

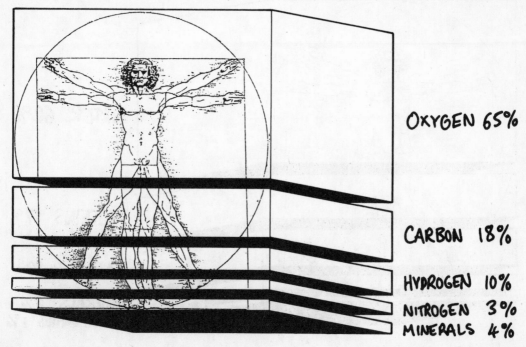

OXYGEN 65%

CARBON 18%

HYDROGEN 10%

NITROGEN 3%

MINERALS 4%

Figure 1.2.1 — *The elements in man*

For example two atoms of hydrogen and one of oxygen make a molecule of water. The skeleton on which the structure of life is built is made of carbon atoms. On to different lengths of carbon chains are added atoms of hydrogen, oxygen and nitrogen to make the three major building blocks of life — proteins, fats and carbohydrates.

The simplest of these substances are carbohydrates, which are made up of atoms of carbon and hydrogen. With the addition of oxygen to the mixture we get the fats, which are important in the membranes surrounding cells, and act as insulation and energy stores. Proteins are made from carbon, oxygen, hydrogen and nitrogen and sometimes sulphur and phosphorus.

Like the rest of life on this planet, we are made up of protein, fat, carbohydrate, minerals and vitamins, and water.

Simple carbohydrates are mainly used as a source of energy — while the very complex carbohydrates (fibre), which are not broken down in digestion, play an important role in maintaining a healthy digestive tract. Protein plays many roles in the body. The enzymes that break down proteins so they can be absorbed into the blood are themselves specialized proteins. Many hormones, which are the chemical messengers of the body's control systems, are proteins; and skin, teeth and bones are all made out of a special protein called collagen. Fats and oils have a number of different functions. They are mainly used as a store of energy, and it is this type of fat which is familiar to most people, as the most visible storage of energy in this way takes place under the skin! Fat acts as insulation against the cold, and it also provides cushioning for delicate organs.

Although only 4% of our bodies consists of minerals, we would not be alive without them. The main structural minerals are calcium, phosphorus and magnesium — all of which are used to make bones. Calcium and magnesium are also important for healthy nerves. The right balance of sodium, potassium and chlorine, in and around our cells, makes sure that we neither dehydrate nor drown in our own fluids, and that our nerves and muscles work well.

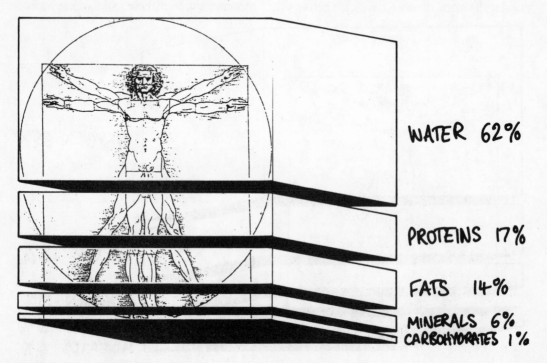

WATER 62%

PROTEINS 17%

FATS 14%

MINERALS 6%
CARBOHYDRATES 1%

Figure 1.2.2 — *Compounds in man*

The trace elements constitute only 0.014% of the elements in the body, yet without them most of the chemical processes that maintain life would grind to a halt. The discovery of the importance of these elements has only come about fairly recently, and the list of minerals that may be important to life in tiny amounts is growing, as more research takes place into this interesting area of human nutrition.

The magical cell

But there is one thing that makes you fundamentally different from just a collection of chemicals and that is life itself. All life forms consist of the smallest 'life unit' — the cell. Some organisms consist of only one cell, like the amoeba. We consist of trillions of cells — brain cells, nerve cells, muscle cells, blood cells and many more — all perfectly organized and connected by chemical and electrical networks of communication. Every day we make and replace billions of cells. Every year a quarter of all our cells are replaced with new cells.

Within each cell, whatever its function, are different 'organelles' involved in making energy, waste disposal and new cell manufacture. All these different activities occur because of enzymes. Enzymes are substances that have the ability to turn one chemical into another. For instance, sugar is turned into water and carbon dioxide by enzymes. This process releases energy and that energy powers the cells in all their different functions.

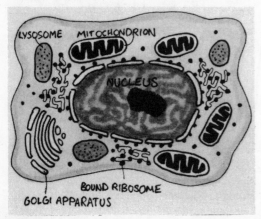

Figure 1.2.3 — *The cell*

Biochemists have known for a long time that by altering the cell's nutrition they can make it work better. In the 1960s, Nobel Prize winner Linus Pauling coined the phrase 'orthomolecular' medicine to describe this science. 'Ortho' means right and what he meant was the science of giving cells the right molecules or nutrients to help them function best. Since we are a collection of highly 'well connected' cells, finding the right mix for our cells is what optimum nutrition is all about. And that depends upon our evolution.

Nutrition and evolution

Like it or not, man is an ape, of class primate, species homo and, we like to think, sapiens. We have been roaming the planet for somewhere in the region of five million years. It is logical to assume that we have evolved to make use of the nutrients available to us during the majority of our evolution while eating a 'caveman diet'.

Man's original diet was very different from the food we eat today. At first we were mainly vegetarian and ate things that grew naturally. Our diet has varied with our developing skills and the changing environments in which we have lived.

When 'Southern Ape' came down from the trees and started to walk on his hind legs, it left him his hands free to carry food back to share with his family in a sheltered camp. His diet was mainly fruit and nuts, and he used a digging stick to find roots and tubers. He would supplement this vegetarian fare with occasional small animals, insects and eggs.

'Handy Man' was a hunter-gatherer, and started making gadgets to help collect food. The females and young gathered fruits, nuts, and vegetables, whilst the males went further afield, first scavenging, and then hunting animals. Although his diet had changed, the actual constituents of his diet, fats, proteins, carbohydrate, vitamins and minerals, hadn't changed much.

'Upright Man' cooked his food on the first barbecue, and this tender meat became a more important part of his diet. The discovery of fire also enabled him to live in colder areas, and to keep predators away. He expanded his range of tools, and as he became more skilful at hunting

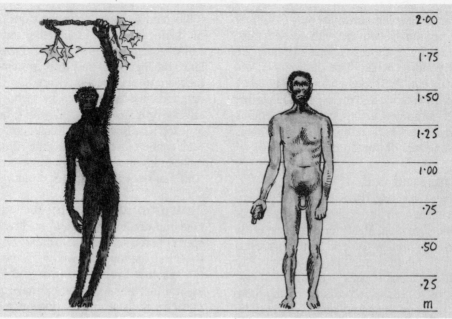

4-2 million years ago
SOUTHERN APE
Ate a largely vegetarian diet using sticks
to dig for roots and vegetables.

2-1 million years ago
HANDY MAN
Made gadgets to collect food and
became a hunter. Discovered fire.

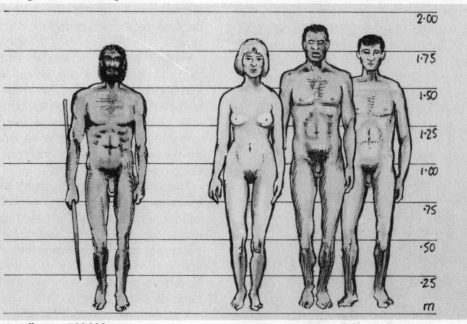

1 million — 500,000 years ago
NEANDERTHAL MAN
Became an intelligent and skilled
hunter, wearing skins to keep warm
in the ice age.

500,000 years ago — today
MODERN MAN
Started to cultivate food and became
a peasant farmer . . .

Figure 1.2.4 — *The evolution of man*

he was able to kill larger animals. 'Neanderthal Man' was able to kill woolly mammoths and bears, and he used their skins to keep himself warm during the ice age.

At the end of the ice age 'Modern Man' hunted the herds of game which he portrayed in cave paintings. As the weather became warmer and wetter the tundra was replaced by grassland, and the grain this yielded was stored until needed, then baked into bread. Grain brought a new emphasis to the diet, and as scattered seed around the camp grew to give a harvest the next year, the first agriculture developed. Man found that he could plan ahead and so was released from the need to collect for his needs every day.

This means that grains of all kinds are a recent addition to our diets. Wheat and barley were first cultivated in the Near East about 9,000 years ago; rice and millet were grown in China 7,000 years ago, and maize was cultivated in Central America 5,000 years ago.

It was not until only the last 200 years, a split second in our history, that our diets changed dramatically. With the Industrial Revolution people began to move to the cities. And through medical advances in treating infectious diseases, populations began to increase.

In this short space of time the world's population shot from one to five billion people. With new demands to feed peole in the cities we learnt how to process foods so they wouldn't deteriorate or be eaten by bugs, not thinking that if a food couldn't support a bug it might not support us. With this new craze for refined, 'pure' food like white flour or white rice, modern man started to develop vitamin, mineral and fibre deficiencies as well as fat, salt and sugar excesses. The incidence of heart disease, cancer, diabetes and a host of other diet-related diseases began to develop within two generations of those first eating the modern day diet. By the 1960s heart disease, cancer and diabetes had reached epidemic proportions and most of the medical research resources were channelled into solving these problems. But solutions involving changes in eating habits are essentially non-profitable for the drug and food industry, so fierce resistance to ideas within nutrition continue to be met.

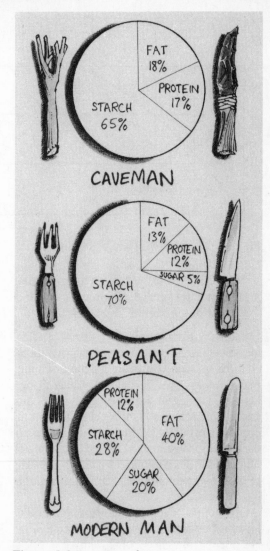

Figure 1.2.5 — *Diet of caveman* vs *peasant* vs *modern man*

Despite this, by the start of the 1980s most western countries began to make positive changes to eating habits and lifestyle and the first signs of a decrease in diet-related diseases began to occur. With this has come a resurgence of interest in the role of nutrition in health both from scientific, medical and public quarters.

Optimum nutrition — the medicine of tomorrow

The doctor of the future will give no medicine

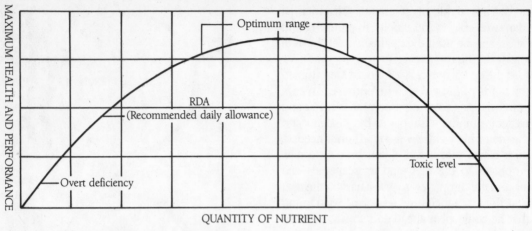

Figure 1.2.6 — *Graph of health vs vitamin intake*

but will interest his patients in the care of the human frame, in diet, and in the cause and prevention of disease. *Thomas Edison.*

Unlike the caveman, who had, like all species, to compete for nutrients and was often left short-changed, modern man can, for the first time, manipulate his environment and wilfully change his diet. While our ancestors' diets may have naturally conformed more closely to our evolutionary design for nutrients, it is only with the rapidly evolving scientific understanding of nutrition that it is becoming increasingly possible to say what optimum nutrition is and to put it into practice.

Optimum nutrition, like health, is not straight-forward to define. It is best illustrated by considering the effects on health of a single vitamin.

When any vitamin is very poorly supplied health is poor and overt deficiency signs develop. As the vitamin dosage is increased a point is reached where overt deficiency signs are no longer present although slight symptoms may still occur. Somewhat above this is where the Recommended Daily Allowance (RDA) is usually set, designed to prevent deficiency symptoms. But only when the amount of the vitamin supplied reaches the top of the graph is nutrition said to be optimum. We can define this as a total lack of associated symptoms of deficiency; or biochemically, as a point where all enzyme systems dependent on this nutrient are functioning optimally; or subjectively, as the point of maximum experienced well-being. As the dosage of most nutrients is increased beyond this point, health will eventually decline until toxicity is reached.

For example, consider this research on rats and vitamin A. When given the equivalent of 1,000iu, rats develop gross deficiency, a loss of vision. At a level of 1,750iu vision returns. When given 5,600iu minimum storage is maintained in the liver. At a further dosage equivalent to 16,800iu maximum growth rate is achieved. But only when 33,600iu are given daily do rats reach maximum production of young. This dose represents thirteen times the RDA of 2,500iu.

So the purpose of optimum nutrition then becomes supplying the optimum levels of all the forty-five or so nutrients upon which we depend by altering our diet and, when necessary, taking vitamin and mineral supplements. However, what is ideal for one person is rarely ideal for another, because nutritional needs depend upon a host of other factors. These include inherited factors, exposure to pollution, stress levels, amount of exercise, age, sex, weight, ability to absorb nutrients, consumption of drugs, alcohol, cigarettes, and other stimulants like coffee, and previous health history.

As you go through each chapter in this book you will discover not only how these factors affect

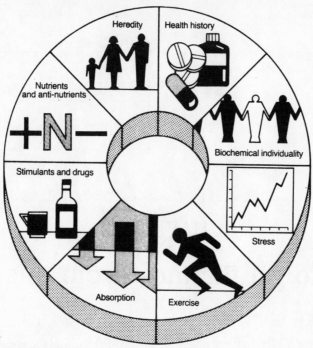

Figure 1.2.7 — *Adjusting factors*

the individual's unique nutritional needs, but also how to take them into account in building your own ideal nutrition programme. The next chapter explains how to get the most from this book.

CHAPTER 1.3

How to get the most from this book

Nutrition is a fascinating subject in its own right and it also has direct relevance to you and your health. For this reason this book is designed not only to give you a solid foundation in nutrition, but also to help you get healthier in the process.

There are two ways of understanding the basics of nutrition. One is to study the human body, how it works and where nutrition fits in. The other is to look at how nutrients work and what they do in the body. Only with a basic understanding of how the body works, and how nutrients function is it possible to understand nutrition in health and disease.

PART 2 explains how the body works by investigating digestion, absorption, metabolism, elimination, the respiratory and cardiovascular system, the nervous and endocrine system and the immune and lymphatic system.

PART 3 examines nutrients. First the macronutrients — fat, protein and carbohydrate, then the micronutrients — vitamins, minerals and essential fatty acids, and finally the anti-nutrients. It then looks at how to balance diet and the pros and cons of special kinds of diets.

PART 4 examines the role optimum nutrition can play in the treatment and prevention of the major diseases of today.

PART 5 looks at the special nutritional needs of the elderly, babies and children, pregnant women and athletes.

PART 6 helps you build your own personal nutrition programme using the Nutrition Programme Questionnaire.

Getting an overview
Each chapter from now on starts with an Overview. This explains, in a nutshell, the contents of the chapter.

Digging deeper
If a particular aspect of this chapter interests you, you may wish to dig deeper. You can do this either by reading the Recommended Further Reading books, or by going to your local library and finding one or more of the Key Research Papers.

Working out your ideal nutrition programme
By the time you reach the end of this book you will have worked out your own ideal diet and supplement programme and will be able to work out diets and supplement programmes suited to an individual's needs.

PART TWO

HOW YOUR BODY WORKS

CHAPTER 2.1

Aiding digestion and absorption

—OVERVIEW—

The purpose of the digestive system is to break down complicated food molecules into simple units that can then be absorbed and utilized by the body. Digestion occurs by the chemical action of enzymes initiating a reaction that breaks the food down into simpler form. Enzymes are sensitive to the acid level in the digestive tract, which can start and stop their release.

Carbohydrate digestion starts in the mouth, where the first carbohydrate digesting enzyme, called an amylase, acts. Protein digestion starts in the stomach, where the first protein digesting enzyme, a proteinase, is released. This enzyme only works in the high acid medium of the stomach. Fat is prepared for digestion by the juices released from the gall bladder, called bile. Fat digestion actually starts in the duodenum, where the fat digesting enzymes, called lipases, are released from the pancreas. The pancreas also releases proteases and amylases, making it the key organ of digestion. Further enzymes are released from the next section of the digestive tract, the jejunum. Once they have acted, proteins have been broken down to amino acids; carbohydrates are now simple sugars; and fats are broken down to glycerol and fatty acids. Absorption then begins.

Sugars, amino acids, fatty acids, glycerol and most vitamins and minerals are absorbed in the small intestine, mainly in the ileum. Water and much of sodium and potassium are absorbed in the large intestine. Indigestible material, called fibre, helps to accelerate the passage of digested material through the large intestine to the rectum, ready for excretion. Bacteria also flourish in the large intestine, completing the final stages of food digestion.

Following absorption, the components of digestion are now ready for one of two fates: *anabolism*, which is the building up of components into body tissues for growth or repair (amino acids are the most important building blocks for this process), and *catabolism*, which is the breaking down of components to produce energy. Energy is required not only for muscular activity, but also for brain activity, digestion and absorption, and anabolism. Simple sugars are the most important source of energy, although fats and indeed amino acids can also be utilized when required. Anabolism and catabolism are collectively known as metabolism.

The mouth

The processes of digestion start, not in the mouth but in the mind. On seeing, smelling or even thinking about food we start to secrete digestive juices which will help to transport and break down food when it arrives. On average we secrete no less than eight litres of digestive juices a day, a large proportion of which is water and most of which is reabsorbed once it has done its job. The first glands that come into action are the

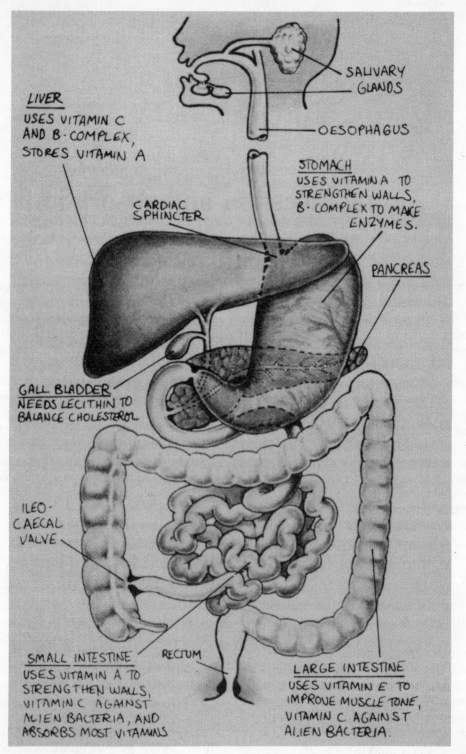

Figure 2.1.1 — *The digestive system*

salivary glands that produce saliva. Saliva also contains the first carbohydrate digesting enzyme, ptyalin. However, ptyalin has little time to act before food is swallowed and travels down the oesophagus entering the stomach through the cardiac sphincter, where the environment is too acidic for ptyalin to work. So the longer a carbohydrate food is chewed the more it will be broken down into simpler sugar units by ptyalin.

The stomach

The stomach is primarily concerned with the digestion of protein, not carbohydrate or fat. Although it does produce a fat splitting enzyme, a lipase, this has negligible effect. Two kinds of cells line the stomach wall. The parietal cells and the chief cells. The parietal cells produce and secrete hydrochloric acid, a process which involves the zinc dependent enzyme carbonic anhydrase, while the chief cells secrete pepsinogen. Hydrochloric acid has the effect of straightening out the curly protein molecules in our food, and then activates pepsinogen, which then becomes pepsin, the first protein digesting enzyme. Pepsin then breaks down protein into smaller chunks called peptides.

Once food leaves the stomach via the pyloric sphincter it is called chyme and has a creamy consistency. It then enters the first and most important part of the small intestine, the duodenum. It is here that digestive juices secreted from the pancreas and gall bladder act on food.

The pancreas

Before the pancreatic enzymes, which travel along the pancreatic duct, can work the environment in the duodenum must be made less acidic. This is done by the release of alkaline salts both from the pancreas and gall bladder. This in turn switches off the pepsin and turns on the pancreatic enzymes.

The pancreas releases: 1) amylases to break down carbohydrates into di-saccharides, 2) proteases, trypsin, chymotrypsin and carboxypeptidase to break down poly-peptides and proteins into di-peptides, 3) lipase to break down fat. However, since these enzymes are all water-based the lipase cannot work well on large globules of fat.

The liver and gall bladder

To get round this problem the gall bladder releases bile into the duodenum in order to emulsify the fat. Emulsification involves turning the large fat molecules into tiny particles with much more surface area of exposed fat for the lipase to work on. Bile is actually produced in the liver and consists of three main ingredients — cholesterol, lecithin and inorganic salts. Bile leaving the liver is largely water, but is further concentrated in the gall bladder. These substances in combination not only allow the fat to become emulsified but have a special way of keeping tiny fat particles separate until absorption takes place. This is called micellization. Each unit of digested fat is incorporated into a structure called a micelle, which repels other micelles thus keeping the fats in solution.

The small intestines

Once the contents of the duodenum enter the next part of the small intestine, the jejunum, most protein is in the form of di-peptides, most carbohydrates are now di-saccharides, and fats are micellized. The intestinal wall continues to secrete digestive enzymes. Di-peptidases are released to break down di-peptides into amino acids and various amylases are released to break down di-saccharides into mono-saccharides.

The predominant types of di-saccharides are maltose, sucrose and lactose. Maltose is the major sugar present in grains. It consists of two glucose molecules and is digested by maltase. Sucrose is sugar as we know it and consists of a glucose and a fructose, or fruit sugar, molecule. It is digested by an enzyme called sucrase. And lactose, or milk sugar, is broken down in galactose and glucose by the enzyme lactase. The most important sugars which are then absorbed are fructose and glucose.

Absorption

Most absorption takes place in the jejunum and ileum, which is the final part of the small intestine, although absorption of some minerals

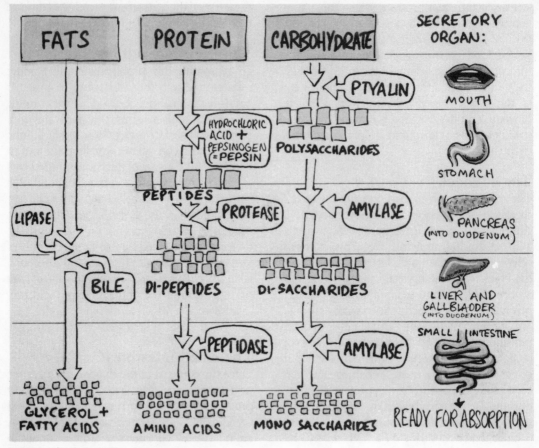

Figure 2.1.2 — *The enzymes of digestion*

and water occurs in the large intestine. Absorption involves the transport of fats, amino acids (and some peptides) and simple sugars out of the digestive tract into the blood or lymphatic vessels. This process is aided by the design of the intestinal wall. Rather than being smooth it consists of millions of tiny folds or protrusions called villi. Within each villus are capillaries (tiny blood vessels) and lymphatic vessels ready to carry out the digested nutrients. These either simply diffuse across the intestinal wall or are actively transported across by a variety of mechanisms. These either involve a pumping mechanism called the sodium pump, or transport via carrier molecules. For example, most of the absorption of amino acids involves carrier molecules dependent on vitamin B_6.

Vitamins do not need to be digested but they do need to be liberated from food in order to be absorbed. Fat soluble vitamins need to be attached to fat molecules for absorption to occur. The absorption of vitamin B_{12} is slightly different. B_{12} must first combine with a protein, called intrinsic factor, which is released in the stomach. Only then can it be absorbed at specific sites in the ileum. Minerals are absorbed both in the small and large intestine.

Fats are eaten in the form of triglycerols. This means there are three fatty acids on a backbone of glycerol, shaped much like the letter E, with each prong being a fatty acid. However, triglycerols can't be absorbed, so the different lipases knock off each fatty acids until only free fatty acids, glycerol or monoglycerols (one fatty acids attached to a backbone of glycerol) are left. These can then be absorbed. But once fat is in the intestinal wall it is then reconstituted into a similar configuration known as a triglyceride and then released into the bloodstream via the lymphatic system.

Metabolism

Most of the amino acids, fats and simple sugars in the bloodstream are then transported to the liver from which some go directly into circulation. Whether they end up in the liver or are supplied directly to muscle cells their fate is basically the same. Amino acids are reconstituted to make proteins, which are then incorporated into cells. Fats are either used for energy, put into storage or are incorporated into cells. For example, cell walls contain fat. Carbohydrates are predominantly used to make energy. The utilization of these nutrients is called metabolism and takes place within every cell. Metabolism itself depends upon nutrients and in the diagram below the major vitamins and minerals involved in the metabolism of protein, fat and carbohydrate are shown.

Catabolism

The process of turning food into energy is called catabolism. Plants produce carbohydrates by using the sun's energy to combine carbon, hydrogen and oxygen. Much in the same way that we burn logs to release the stored energy as heat, our cells oxidize carbohydrates to release the stored energy. This energy is used to power the chemical processes which we know of as life, and to provide heat. But if we were to 'burn' carbohydrate the result would be a sudden release of heat and no energy for body processes. It is as if the energy in carbohydrate is in one currency, and the kind of energy we need to power cells is in another. The gradual release of energy in a form that the body can use happens through a series of chemical reactions that have taken half a century for chemists to unravel and about which there are still many mysteries. The series of chemical reactions can be seen in three distinct sections: glycolysis, the citric acid (or Krebs) cycle and the electron transfer pathway.

The first part of the process, glycolysis, involves the processing of glucose from diet, or glycogen, the form in which glucose is stored in muscles, into pyruvic acid. This releases a small amount of energy for work by the body. It also is not dependent on the presence of oxygen. For example, if you were to do a short sprint and ended up panting, the demand on your muscles to produce energy without having an adequate supply of oxygen would have meant the processing of glucose to pyruvic acid anaerobically. Under these circumstances pyruvic acid is then converted to lactic acid, which can build up in the muscles with anaerobic exercise and makes them feel stiff.

The presence of sufficient oxygen, supplied by

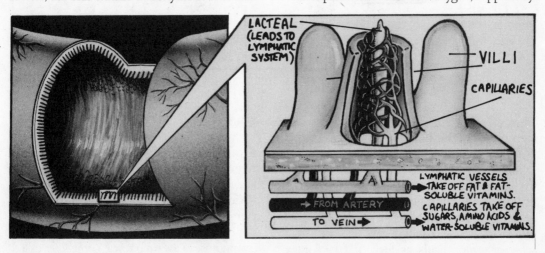

Figure 2.1.3 — *Detail and section of the villi*

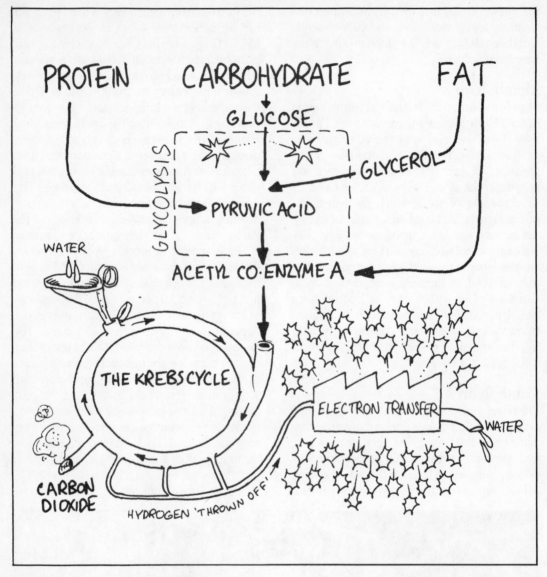

Figure 2.1.4 — *The major metabolic pathways*

breathing, and then transported in the form of haemoglobin in the blood, allows more energy to be generated during glycolysis and pyruvic acid is converted into acetyl coenzyme A. This step involves thiamine, vitamin B_1.

When there are insufficient supplies of glucose or glycogen, for example during a fast or after twenty miles of a marathon, we can use fatty acids or amino acids as fuel. In fact, some muscles, e.g. the heart, prefer fatty acids to glucose

as fuel. These are converted into acetyl coenzyme A which then shares the same metabolic pathway as carbohydrate. The production of this key metabolite depends upon vitamin B_5, pantothenic acid.

Acetyl coenzyme A then enters a cycle of chemical reactions known as the Krebs cycle, after Hans Krebs, who discovered it in the 1950s. The purpose of the Krebs cycle, sometimes called the citric acid cycle, is to pass hydrogen atoms into another pathway, called the electron transfer pathway. The by-product of the Krebs cycle is carbon dioxide.

The electron transfer pathway depends upon vitamins B_2, B_3 and C and it is along this pathway that most of our energy is produced. The end product of the electron transfer pathway is water. So, overall, we can write the energy equation as:

GLUCOSE + OXYGEN → WATER + CARBON DIOXIDE + ENERGY

or in the language of chemistry

$$C_6H_{12}O_6 + {_6}O_2 \rightarrow {_6}H_2O + {_6}CO_2 + ATP$$

But what is the energy that is released? The process of glycolysis (in the presence of oxygen) gives rise to four units of a highly reactive substance, adenosine triphosphate (ATP). The electron transfer pathway gives rise to a further 34 units of ATP. ATP is the form of energy used to power muscles and other body processes that create enzymes, build up protein, and carry out the work of the human body. This energy is released by converting ATP into adenosine diphosphate (ADP) and a phosphate molecule. The equation looks like this:

ATP → ADP + P + MUSCULAR ACTIVITY

Throughout these processes heat is also lost, so that for each unit of energy derived from glucose, 38 per cent is lost as heat, which then heats the body, and 42 per cent is released as ATP to power cells. This is why we get hot when using lots of energy as in exercise. For the muscles to react, calcium and magnesium must be present in and around muscle cells. For the transport of oxygen we need iron. And for the transport of glucose from the blood to the cell we need chromium.

Anabolism

Some of the energy released from catabolism is used to help build new cells. This process is called anabolism. Cells are predominantly made out of protein. When a cell needs to be built or replaced (for example when exercising new muscle, cells are being built up to develop stronger muscles to cope with the exercise) the body must select the appropriate ingredients from neighbouring tissues, break down products of old cells or from the bloodstream. The liver not only releases individual amino acids into circulation but also reconstitutes and releases proteins for use as building material for new cells. There is also a process called transamination which allows one amino acid to be converted into another (although only certain amino acids can be converted into certain others). Through a complex process involving RNA and DNA the body reconstitutes these amino acids and other building material to make new cells.

Elimination

The substances that need to be eliminated from the body can be divided into four categories:

1) End products of metabolism. This includes carbon dioxide, water from carbohydrate metabolism, and urea, uric acid and ammonia from protein metabolism.
2) Indigestible constituents of food. This includes fibre, and indigestible proteins.
3) Excessive levels of nutrients. This includes sodium, potassium, calcium and magnesium, which are excreted to maintain the right balance of these 'electrolytes' involved in muscle and nerve transmission.
4) Toxic material. This includes certain food additives, pollutants, and breakdown products of alcohol.

These unwanted substances can be primarily eliminated via the kidneys, lungs and skin (explained in the next chapter) or via the gastrointestinal tract.

The large intestine

Once food has been digested and the nutritional contents absorbed what is left passes into the large intestine or colon through the ileo-caecal valve situated near the right hip close to the appendix. This valve is particularly important in that the colon contains on average 3lbs of bacteria many of which should not be present in the small intestine. The main purpose of the large intestine is to absorb water and produce faeces which are then moved along the colon by means of a peristaltic movement of the muscles surrounding the colon. Some absorption of minerals also occurs. Faecal matter collects in the rectal area ready for excretion.

Problems and diseases of the digestive system

Many things can go wrong with digestion and absorption, most of which are the consequence of faulty nutrition. Here is a brief description of the commonest problems, their causes and nutritional remedies.

Achlorhydria is an insufficiency in the production of hydrochloric acid in the stomach. In its severest form it is a very serious condition in that protein cannot be broken down. It can be caused by a lack of zinc, in which case zinc supplementation will help. Indigestion is the major symptom.

Candida Albicans (also called thrush) is a yeast-like organism that can thrive in the gastrointestinal tract when beneficial bacteria levels are low. It may cause tiny white spots in the mouth, or anal itching. A diet low in sugar and fat and high in fibre, and rich in beneficial bacteria provided by yogurt or supplements like lactobacillus acidophilus, makes it less easy for this organism to thrive.

Coeliac disease is a sensitivity to gluten, a protein found predominantly in wheat. It cause atrophy of the villi and hence causes malabsorption. Symptoms include signs of malnourishment and loss of weight despite adequate nutrition. It is thought that other food allergies may also damage the intestinal tract.

Colitis is an inflammation of the wall of the colon. Ulcers may form, which is called ulcerative colitis. A symptom is blood in faeces. It is primarily caused by a low fibre, high meat, milk or egg diet, all highly mucus-forming, resulting in compacted faeces, and a swollen or inflamed colon. Although a high fibre, predominantly raw food, diet is helpful changes should be made gradually.

Constipation is one of the commonest 'illnesses' in the western world. Although it has come to mean discomfort caused by infrequency of bowel motion, it in fact refers to faecal matter that is compacted and heavy, rather than loosely formed, light faecal matter which is associated with a healthy diet. A diet deriving fibre from vegetables, whole cereals, beans and pulses and fruit, and not excessive in meat, milk or eggs usually relieves this problem.

Diarrhoea can be caused by an infection in the gut (see gastroenteritis) or a muscular contraction of the colon as a result of irritation caused by old faecal matter, coffee, spicy food or a food allergen. Since diarrhoea causes a loss of fluids sufficient water must be drunk. Loose bowel motions, not diarrhoea, are consistent with a diet high in fibre and are no cause for concern.

Diverticulosis describes the formation of pockets or pouches in the colon as a result of build up of pressure from a low fibre diet. If these 'diverticula' become inflamed, which they are prone to do since faecal matter cannot pass along easily, this is called diverticulitis.

Duodenal Ulcer is an ulcer normally in the first part of the duodenum beside the pyloric sphincter. It may be caused by excessive stomach acid (see overacidity) or a lack of vitamin A which helps strengthen mucus membranes. A high alkaline-forming diet plus supplementation of vitamin A is recommended.

Flatulence (either bloatedness or excessive wind) is produced during the bacterial fermentation of fibre. It can result from incomplete digestion providing bacteria with extra nourishment. The bacteria produce gas which results in flatulence. Reasons for indigestion should then be explored. Some foods, for example beans, contain relatively indigestible proteins and hence cause flatulence.

Food Allergy can cause intestinal irritation, resulting in diarrhoea and hence indigestion. It is likely that prolonged ingestion of allergens may cause atrophy of the villi as seen in coeliac disease. Milk and grain (particularly wheat) allergy are the most common. Milk allergy should be suspected in babies with colic. Breastfed babies can react to an allergen eaten by the mother.

Gallstones can be either an improper build up of calcium crystals or cholesterol, either in the gall bladder or in the bile duct. This can cause restricted flow of bile, resulting in impaired fat digestion and jaundice. There is some evidence that cholesterol gallstones can be broken down by dietary intervention. Obviously a low fat, low cholesterol diet is recommended.

Gastroenteritis refers to inflammation of the gastrointestinal tract caused by infection. This is usually the result of food poisoning or gastric 'flu'. It is best not to eat, or to eat easily digested foods, until it is gone.

Irritable Bowel Syndrome refers to a problem of frequent and sudden defaecation, often involving diarrhoea or constipation and diarrhoea. In some cases food allergy is suspected. It often occurs in anxious people and may have a psychological basis.

Malabsorption is to be suspected in people who are losing weight despite eating a nutritious diet. It may be the result of indigestion, a food allergy, or a 'gunked up' intestinal tract. The treatment depends upon which cause is suspected.

Overacidity results from an excessive production of hydrochloric acid and produces heartburn and indigestion. Indigestion is often wrongly attributed to overacidity. But indigestion can also be caused by under acidity. Since antacids can also trigger acid production in someone with low acid levels, they provide relief for both situations. A diet high in protein may induce overacidity. Stress is also associated with this condition. A diet high in alkaline-forming foods is recommended.

Pancreatic Insufficiency describes an inability of the pancreatic cells to produce digestive enzymes. This can occur due to poor nutrition since B_6 and zinc, and probably other B vitamins, are required to make these enzymes work. Supplementation with B_6 and zinc is obviously recommended and so is supplementation with pancreatic enzymes to allow digestion to be complete. Digestive enzyme supplements may not be required once the pancreas returns to normal function.

Peptic (stomach) Ulcer is the same as duodenal ulcer except it occurs usually in the lower portion of the stomach which is more acidic.

CHAPTER 2.2

Improving circulation and respiration

—OVERVIEW—

For life to occur four major elements are required, carbon, hydrogen, nitrogen and oxygen. The first three are primarily supplied from food. Oxygen is supplied from air. Air enters the lungs, filling up balloon-like sacks called alveoli. From there oxygen passes into the blood stream and then to the heart, which pumps the oxygen to every cell in the body. The blood also contains fats, proteins, sugars, vitamins, minerals and other vital chemicals needed to nourish and regulate body processes in the cells of which we are made. So the blood is our major transport system. It also transports unwanted material, like carbon dioxide back to the lungs, or waste products of metabolism to the kidneys.

Vessels which carry freshly oxygenated blood are called arteries. These turn into arterioles and later capillaries, which are thin and permeable allowing delivery and collection of substances from the cell. The artery then becomes a vein, carrying carbon dioxide-rich blood back to the lungs for re-oxygenation.

The kidneys are designed to filter out unwanted substances from the blood. Blood enters the kidneys at high pressure and fluid, containing the waste products of metabolism in addition to glucose and useful mineral salts, is forced out of the artery into the kidney nephron. The kidney then selectively reabsorbs some materials in preference to others.

The nitrogenous end products of protein metabolism, urea and uric acid, are not reabsorbed, and when diluted with water to protect the rest of the excretory system from this strong acid, form urine. Many vitamins and minerals and glucose are reabsorbed. When glucose is found in the urine this is a marker of diabetes. The kidneys also control the water balance in the body by manipulating the minerals sodium and potassium and hormones governing their balance. Since we are 62% water maintaining water balance is crucial.

The useful substances are therefore reabsorbed and the waste products pass along the ureter to the bladder for excretion via the urethra.

The respiratory system provides us with the most essential nutrient of all — oxygen. Without it we cannot live for more than five minutes. However oxygen is also one of the most dangerous substances in our bodies. To understand oxygen let us first return through our evolutionary past to the beginning of life itself.

The first simple cells were probably anaerobic algae and bacteria. Not only did these life forms not consume oxygen, they actually produced it as a waste product. The initial quantities produced reacted with metals like iron to produce oxides or rust. However, when all the suitable metals had been oxidized, oxygen began to accumulate. In these early days oxygen was a threat to life itself as it was toxic to these early life forms. Fortunately a crisis was averted,

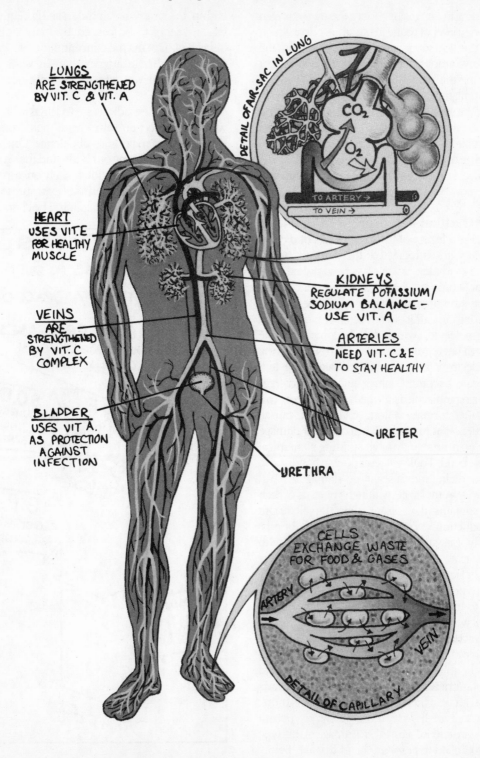

Figure 2.2.1 — *The respiratory and circulatory system*

according to one major current theory, by oxygen forming a layer of ozone in the atmosphere which had the added advantage of preventing the excessive amount of dangerous ultraviolet light reaching the planet's surface. This slowed the acculumlation of oxygen down sufficiently to allow the evolution of oxygen-utilizing bacteria that evolved into animal life. The original anaerobic bacteria accustomed themselves to the presence of oxygen and developed into plant life, and a balanced and harmonious system was achieved.

Free radicals

However, a legacy of the toxic effects of oxygen remain with us today. For the damage caused by free-oxidizing radicals has been linked with cancer, coronary heart disease, rheumatoid arthritis and premature ageing. So, what is a free-oxidizing radical? It is a molecule or radical (part of a molecule) which has become unstable through having an unpaired electron. In pairing this electron with another molecule, the first molecule becomes stable, but a second free-oxidizing molecule is formed. This process can continue, forming a long chain that causes destruction at each step. The particular damage done is invariably through splitting a chemical double bond. Thus wherever double bonds exist, free-oxidizing radicals will do damage.

The DNA molecule, within the nucleus of each cell, contains the master plans for all future reproduction. It contains many double bonds. Clearly if its structure is damaged its ability to replicate accurately will be impaired, which is a major factor in premature ageing. An even more serious possibility is that the damaged DNA will lead to mutations responsible for cancer.

Cell walls are made of unsaturated fatty acids which contain double bonds and are thus susceptible to free radical damage. Strong cell walls, with the ability to regulate the movement in and out of nutrients, are one of the primary criteria for health on a biochemical level. What is more, weak cell walls are more likely to permit mutation, and hence cancer. Damage of this type is also linked to coronary heart disease. Before cholesterol-containing plaque can build up

within the artery a 'binding site' is required, which seems to be caused by free-oxidizing radical damage. As the concentration of oxygen is much higher in arteries than in veins, this would explain why atheromas only occur in arteries.

If free-oxidizing radicals are so lethal, what can we do to protect ourselves from their damage? There are two main lines of defence. One is to prevent them entering our body, and the second involves breaking them down safely once inside. One of the commonest forms of exposure to free radicals is atmospheric pollution. The chemicals

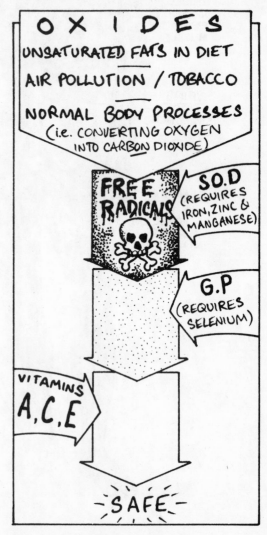

Figure 2.2.2 — *Anti-oxidants*

found in smog, pesticides, car exhaust fumes all produce high levels of free-oxidizing radicals. Radiation can have this effect also. Foods are not free either. For instance caffeine contains a chemical, xanthine, which is then broken down to produce oxides. However, maybe the most dangerous food source is rancid unsaturated fats. On exposure to heat or light the double bond in polyunsaturated fats is oxidized to provide the starting point for a chain reaction of free-oxidizing radicals. Thus unsaturated oils and fats should be kept in a refrigerator and not used for cooking. Butter or olive oil are much safer options where heat is involved.

However careful one is, free-oxidizing radicals will always find their way into the body, and so must be safely metabolized. This is done in two stages. The first requires enzymes to break them down into stable and harmless compounds. The most important anti-oxidant enzymes are two forms of superoxide dismutase, one containing zinc and copper, the other manganese, glutathione peroxidase (which is selenium based) and glutathione reductase.

The second form of defence is based on vitamins E, A and C. A and E are fat soluble and so provide the main anti-oxidant protection within the cell wall. Vitamin C is water soluble and acts as a roaming scavenger complementing the effects of vitamins E and A and occurring in high concentrations within the brain, lungs and adrenal glands.

So oxygen really has a ubiquitous nature within the body. It provides the force for all energy producing reactions, yet its very reactivity which permits this to happen is the basis of very damaging chemicals.

The lungs

Oxygen, our most vital nutrient, although present in food, is predominantly supplied to us through the lungs. The air passes along the trachea down the bronchus into one of three lobes of either lung. There the air fills up balloon-like structures called the alveoli. The alveoli pass oxygen into the blood and take up carbon dioxide which we then exhale. Most people use less than a third of their available lung capacity in normal breathing. The remainder is available for use at times when the body needs a good supply of oxygen, such as in exercise. One of the markers of ageing is a loss of elasticity of the lung tissue. This elasticity is maintained by the intercellular glue, collagen, which is dependent on an adequate supply of vitamin C. Since the lungs are also exposed to alien substances, like viruses, that we'd rather didn't get inside us, maintaining a strong lung wall is helped by adequate intake of vitamin A. Both vitamin C, A and E are also anti-oxidants which can protect the cells in the lungs walls from becoming damaged from inhaled oxides, the result of polluted or smoky air. These can trigger off lung cancer, which is discussed in more detail in Chapter 4.2.

The blood

Blood, of which we have five litres, is red because of a special substance in red blood cells called haemoglobin which carries oxygen to each body cell. Haemoglobin is dependent on the mineral iron. When iron levels are low haemoglobin levels will also drop. As well as transporting oxygen and carbon dioxide the blood transports fats, simple sugars, amino acids and proteins, enzymes, hormones, vitamins, minerals and waste products.

It also contains antibodies which ward off foreign invaders like bugs or allergens. These are discussed in more detail in Chapter 2.4.

The heart

The blood reaches every cell in the body because it is pumped around the body by our strongest muscle, the heart. The heart beats with military regularity over 1,500 times a day, or 600,000 times a year and 45 million times in a lifetime. More than any other part of the body it needs a good supply of oxygen.

Arteries and veins

Oxygen is supplied to the heart muscle and indeed every muscle along arteries, that lead into arterioles, then capillaries which are only one cell thick. When the capillaries have given off their nutrients and collected waste materials they lead into veins which return to the lungs in order

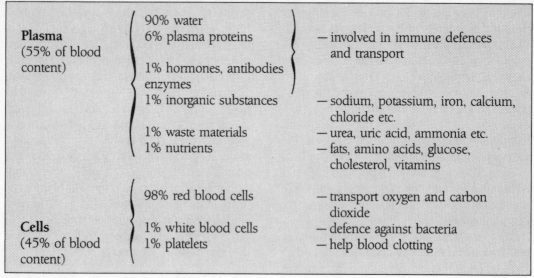

Plasma (55% of blood content)	90% water	— involved in immune defences and transport
	6% plasma proteins	
	1% hormones, antibodies enzymes	
	1% inorganic substances	— sodium, potassium, iron, calcium, chloride etc.
	1% waste materials	— urea, uric acid, ammonia etc.
	1% nutrients	— fats, amino acids, glucose, cholesterol, vitamins
Cells (45% of blood content)	98% red blood cells	— transport oxygen and carbon dioxide
	1% white blood cells	— defence against bacteria
	1% platelets	— help blood clotting

Chart 2.2.1 — *What the blood consists of*

to re-oxygenate the blood and release carbon dioxide into the lungs. Blood also passes through the kidneys which filter out undesirable substances.

The major causes of death in the western world are the diseases of the arteries. These are discussed in full in chapter 4.1. The link to faulty nutrition has been clearly established as a major cause of heart and artery disease. How to reduce the risk of these diseases is also known, but involves dietary and lifestyle changes about which many people are ignorant and others unwilling to make. But how do you know if you have a high risk of cardiovascular disease? Two simple indicators are your pulse and blood pressure.

Your pulse and blood pressure

Your pulse and blood pressure are two simple monitors of the health of your heart and cardiovascular system.

Your pulse is a measure of how often your heart needs to beat to get all the blood round your body. A strong heart may only need to beat 60 times or less a minute, while a weak heart may need to beat 75 times or more a minute. Both exercise and good nutrition reduce pulse rate. The ideal pulse rate is below 70 although the average pulse rate is often higher than this.

How to take your pulse

Your pulse can be found inside the bony protuberance of the thumb side of your wrist. Alternatively you can take it by place your fingertips on the side of your neck. You will, of course, need a watch with a second hand.

It is often useful to measure your pulse during exercise as a measure of how hard you are working the cardiovascular system. As your heart

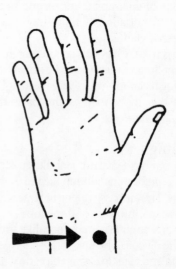

Figure 2.2.3 — *Taking your pulse*

Age	Maximum heart rate	80% of maximum exercise pulse	75% of maximum for heart disease patients
20	200	160	150
22	198	158	148
24	196	157	147
26	194	155	145
28	194	154	144
30	190	152	143
32	189	151	142
34	187	150	140
36	186	149	140
38	184	147	138
40	182	146	137
45	179	143	134
50	175	140	131
55	171	137	128
60	160	128	120
65+	150	120	113

Chart 2.2.2 — *Your ideal exercising pulse rate*

rate can reduce quickly after stopping exercise your exercising pulse should be done only for six seconds. So if you are jogging, start running on the spot as you find your pulse and the second hand on your watch, then stop and take your pulse for six seconds. Multiply this by ten to give your pulse rate per minute. This is what it should be.

Your blood pressure

Your blood pressure is a measure of the pressure your blood exerts as it flows through your arteries. It has two parts. As your heart beats blood is pushed through the arteries at a maximum pressure. This is the first, or systolic reading. Between each beat the pressure falls and reaches a minimum just before the next beat. This is the second or diastolic reading.

A normal blood pressure reading is 120/80. High blood-pressure is a risk factor for heart disease. With a poor diet and lack of exercise blood pressure will gradually rise with age. A reading of 160/95 or above warrants attention. The easiest way to monitor your blood-pressure is to ask your doctor to measure it for you.

Kidneys

The kidneys, situated in the small of the back, either side of the spine, are our filtration plant. Each day they filter 900 litres of blood, helping to maintain the right balance of nutrients within the body. The kidneys are also our primary source for excreting excess water, sodium and the end products of protein metabolism. The body is constantly breaking down excess or unwanted amino acids in a process called deamination. This produces ammonia and urea, both nitrogen compounds. When fat is used to provide energy we may produce ketones. Excess of these substances must be excreted via the kidneys. An excess of purines in the diet, rich in yeast, sardines, shellfish, roe and organ meats, coupled with an inability to get rid of them, causes a build up of uric acid which then forms sodium urate crystals which embed in fingers and toes and cause joint pain, inflammation and stiffness. This is called gout and may be helped by reducing purine rich foods and keeping protein intake adequate but not excessive.

But the most important substance for elimination by the kidneys is water. The chart

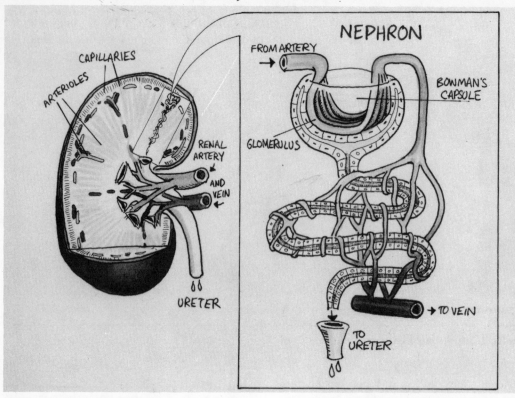

Figure 2.2.4 — *The kidneys*

below shows the balance between intake and output of water. Notice how much water is created from catabolism, the production of energy primarily from glucose and fat. This is called metabolic water. Also notice how much water is lost through the skin. But the predominant loss is via the kidneys.

Intake	ml/day
Drunk	1200
In food	1000
Metabolically produced	350
Total	2550
Output	
Skin and lungs (evaporation)	900
Sweat	50
Faeces	100
Urine	1500
Total	2550

Chart 2.2.3 — *Water balance in man*

The process of filtration takes place in the nephrons of the kidneys producing urine which then passes along the two ureters into the bladder and from there along the urethra for urination. Once urine has left the kidneys the rest is effectively plumbing. So how do the kidneys work?

The blood enters the kidneys via the renal artery and travels along tiny arteries which then divide into fifty or so capillary tufts collectively known as the glomerulus. This construction creates pressure which forces part of the contents of the blood, the plasma, through the capillaries into the mouth of the kidney nephron called the Bowman's capsule. The length of each nephron, of which there are many, is surrounded by capillaries leading back to arteries. These can either secrete substances into the nephron or reabsorb contents from it. The remaining contents travel along to what is called the pelvis of the kidneys and into the ureter. The capillaries then lead to the vein, taking blood back into circulation. Some substances are readily reabsorbed, namely glucose, most of the water, sodium chloride and other salts, amino acids and vitamin C; some are less well reabsorbed, namely potassium; some are very poorly absorbed, namely urea, phosphates, uric acid and ammonia; and some are not reabsorbed at all, namely creatinine and sulphates.

But obviously these rates of reabsorption are not fixed otherwise why would it be that urine production increases when more water is drunk, and that, whether you eat a large amount of salt or a little, the sodium level in the blood stays relatively constant? Also, what happens when, as in diabetes, glucose appears in the urine?

Well, in the case of most substances there is a limit to just how much can be reabsorbed. In the case of glucose, concentration of glucose in the blood can double before any glucose will be found in the urine. But eventually maximum reabsorption capacity is reached and sugar appears in the urine. This is easily tested.

Salt

Let's now consider salt. The chart below shows how salt intake matches salt output. Salt (sodium chloride) intake varies anywhere from 20 grams for a 'saltaholic' to 0.05 grams for someone on a very low salt diet. The present estimated average intake of salt is 12 grams per day. This is far in excess of our needs. The World Health Organization recommend an intake of 5 grams and the NACNE report recommends a reduction of three grams a day, which has been shown to bring down blood pressure in susceptible individuals.

Intake	Gms/day
Food	10.5
Output	
Sweat	0.25
Faeces	0.25
Urine	10.0
Total	10.5

Chart 2.2.4 — *Salt balance in man*

The kidneys also have to eliminate other substances like heavy metals. If they work too hard for too long they may begin to malfunction. When nephrons become inflamed and die off this is called nephritis. For such people low protein and low salt diets are recommended.

CHAPTER 2.3

Balancing nerves and hormones

—OVERVIEW—

All the processes of the body, from breathing to digestion, from walking to talking, are carefully controlled and co-ordinated events. The control of these functions is carried out by two body systems: the nervous system and the endocrine system.

The nervous system consists of millions of nerve cells, the majority of which are in the brain, which pass electrical messages by means of chemical changes that occur in the cells. These messages can cause a muscle cell to contract, transporting visual information from the eye to the brain, or many other forms of direct communication. The nervous system is divided into two parts: the central nervous system and the autonomic nervous system. The central nervous system is the means by which we can turn thoughts into actions. For example, the decision to walk is mediated by the central nervous system. The autonomic nervous system controls automatic body functions like digestion and breathing.

The endocrine system effects control by releasing more long acting chemical messengers called hormones. These are produced in endocrine glands. Hormones are transported around the body in the bloodstream and can turn on or off different chemical reactions. The hormone adrenalin, produced in the adrenal gland, gets us ready to fight or take flight. This is called the stress reaction. The hormone oestrogen causes secondary sexual characteristics in adolescent girls. The control of hormone release is governed by feedback loops, called homeostatic mechanisms, between endocrine glands. To give an example of homeostasis, the master gland, the pituitary, releases thyroid-stimulating hormone which stimulates the thyroid gland to produce thyroxine, speeding up the rate of metabolism. When circulating thyroid levels are high enough, this in turn tells the pituitary to stop producing thyroid-stimulating hormone.

In the past decade a new type of hormone-like substance, called a prostaglandin, has been discovered to influence body chemistry. These prostaglandins are made from essential fatty acids. This important discovery has renewed interest in fats. (This is covered in Chapter 3.4.)

Also involved with control is the immune system. This system is designed to protect us from viruses, bacteria and unhealthy cells, like cancer cells. The immune system is covered in chapter 4.2.

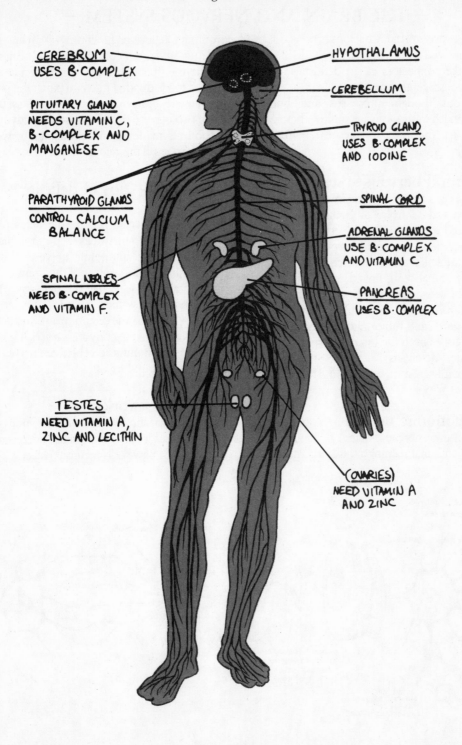

CEREBRUM
USES B·COMPLEX

HYPOTHALAMUS

CEREBELLUM

PITUITARY GLAND
NEEDS VITAMIN C,
B·COMPLEX AND
MANGANESE

THYROID GLAND
USES B·COMPLEX
AND IODINE

PARATHYROID GLANDS
CONTROL CALCIUM
BALANCE

SPINAL CORD

ADRENAL GLANDS
USE B·COMPLEX
AND VITAMIN C

SPINAL NERVES
NEED B·COMPLEX
AND VITAMIN F.

PANCREAS
USES B·COMPLEX

TESTES
NEED VITAMIN A,
ZINC AND LECITHIN

(OVARIES)
NEED VITAMIN A
AND ZINC

Figure 2.3.1 — *The control system*

—THE BRAIN AND NERVOUS SYSTEM—

The brain consists of many millions of nerve cells, cross-connected to each other by around 10,000 tentacle-like connectors called dendrites. The electrical messages that pass between these cells include our thought processes and body feedback mechanisms, causing minute chemical changes in the level of neurotransmitter substances.

The central nervous system

The nervous system is concerned with the integration and control of all bodily functions. It is divided into the Central Nervous System (CNS) and the Autonomic Nervous System.

The central nervous system consists of the brain and spinal cord, linked to a peripheral network of sensory nerve fibres (which carry messages from tissues and organs to the brain or spinal cord) and motor nerve fibres (which carry messages from the brain and spinal cord to the tissues and organs). It is the CNS that allows us to make muscular movements and to process visual information.

The autonomic nervous system

The autonomic nervous system is concerned primarily with maintaining a stable internal environment. It governs functions which are normally not under our control, such as breathing, digestion, temperature regulation, heart rate and so on. It too is divided into two parts: the parasympathetic and sympathetic nervous system. These two oppose each other so the activity of the body is made up of the balance between these two parts of the autonomic nervous system.

The brain — 2lbs of delicate software

The higher control centres of the different aspects of the nervous system are located in the brain. For example, the autonomic nervous system includes the control centres of the brain called the midbrain, pons and medulla oblongata. The central nervous system includes the largest portion of the brain, the cerebrum, in which 90% of all nerve cells in the body are located. It is here that the intercommunication between nerve cells is at a maximum.

How nerves work

Intercommunication within this network provides the basis for all our thoughts, actions and emotions. The nerve cells (neurons) differ widely

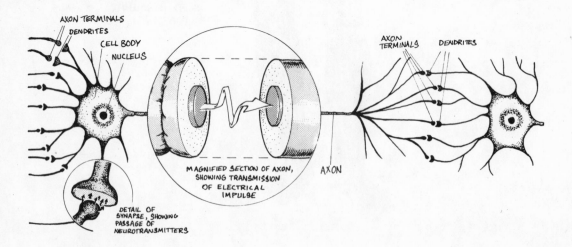

Figure 2.3.2 — *Nerve transmission*

in shape and form but have a similar function. They consist of a cell body containing the nucleus, one or more dendrites which receive the incoming signals, and a branching axon, which transmits a signal onto the next neuron. Information is transferred along each neuron by means of an electrical impulse caused first by an influx of sodium ions, closely followed by a discharge of potassium ions. Once reaching the end of an axon, the impulse needs to cross a small gap, known as a synapse, to the next dendrite. Despite being only in the order of five thousandths of a millimetre, in most cases this is too far for an impulse to jump.

To help transfer the message a group of substances called neurotransmitters are released at the end of each axon and stimulate a nerve impulse in the next dendrite. But not all neurotransmitters help this process. Some are *excitatory*, that is, they are stimulated into a response by the incoming message, and some are *inhibitory*, that is, the signal discourages the neuron from firing.

So whether a neuron fires depends not only on the total number of signals received from other neurons, but also of the net effect of the neurotransmitters. Neurotransmitters play a vital role in regulating the whole nervous system, and many require specific vitamins for their manufacture.

—THE ENDOCRINE SYSTEM—

The endocrine system forms a network of glands that secrete hormones. These hormones control many of the processes that happen inside us. Hormones can be made out of protein, like insulin, or predominantly out of fat, like cortisone. These are called steroid hormones. Most hormones are themselves controlled by means of feedback. An example of this feedback mechanism is seen by examining the pituitary.

The pituitary
Called the master gland because of its overall control, the pituitary governs the functioning of the thyroid gland, the adrenal glands, and the sex glands. It is divided into two parts: the posterior and anterior pituitary. The anterior pituitary produces thyroid stimulating hormone (TSH), adreno-corticotrophic hormone (ACTH), and gonadotrophic hormone which stimulate respectively the thyroid, adrenal cortex and sex glands. These glands in response produce thyroxine, cortisone, oestrogen and progesterone, or in the male testosterone.

As the level of these hormones rises, that instructs the pituitary to stop producing its stimulating hormones. The anterior pituitary also produces somatotrophin or growth hormone, which

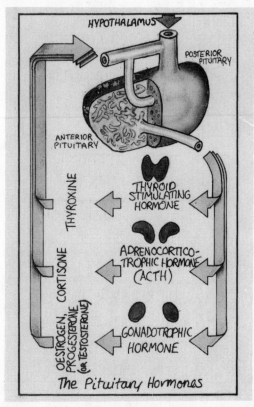

Figure 2.3.3 — *The endocrine glands and hormones*

is mainly active in childhood to stimulate growth, and prolactin which is released in the mother after birth to stimulate milk production. The posterior pituitary produces anti-diuretic hormone (ADH) which helps regulate water balance in the body by helping the kidneys to retain body fluid. It also produces oxytocin which stimulates muscle contractions during and after giving birth.

The stress reaction and the adrenals

Our ability to deal with stress is also under the control of the endocrine system. Stress induces a series of reactions known as the 'fight or flight syndrome' since their accumulative effect prepares the body for physical action and energy expenditure. The initial immediate effect occurs because the brain stimulates one part of the adrenal glands, the adrenal medulla, to produce adrenalin. Adrenalin raises blood sugar levels by causing the liver to break down and release sugar stores. Blood pressure and heartbeat increase to help get the sugar from the blood to the cells. Breathing is stimulated, helping increase available oxygen. Digestion stops and even the blood becomes stickier to help coagulation in case of a cut.

In the long term, stress also stimulates the pituitary to release ACTH, which stimulates the adrenal cortex. This then releases a group of hormones called the corticoids. The glucocorticoids further help make glucose available to cells; while the mineralocorticoids help retain sodium, needed in nerve and muscle transmission.

Maintaining blood sugar balance

Both the release of adrenalin and the glucocorticoids (like cortisone, which incidentally is a powerful anti-inflammatory substance) raise blood sugar levels. This increase triggers the pancreas to produce insulin, a hormone which helps transport glucose into the cells. The liver releases a substance called glucose tolerance factor (based on chromium, B_3 and three amino acids) which also aids glucose transport to the cells. When the blood sugar level drops too low, another pancreatic hormone glucagon, can be released to stimulate the breakdown of liver glycogen to glucose, fat and protein to provide energy.

Once the blood sugar level stays low this stimulates the hypothalamus in the brain and we feel hungry. Since most stress factors are mental, emotional or nutritional and do not require a physical response, the glucose which has been made available is often not required and is returned to storage as fat or glycogen. It is this frequent overstimulation, or the excessive consumption of sugar that leads to problems of obesity and to an inability to maintain an even blood sugar level. In its worst form this results in diabetes. These subjects are discussed in detail in Chapter 4.6.

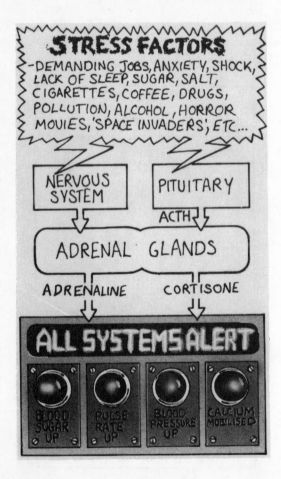

Figure 2.3.4 — *The stress reaction*

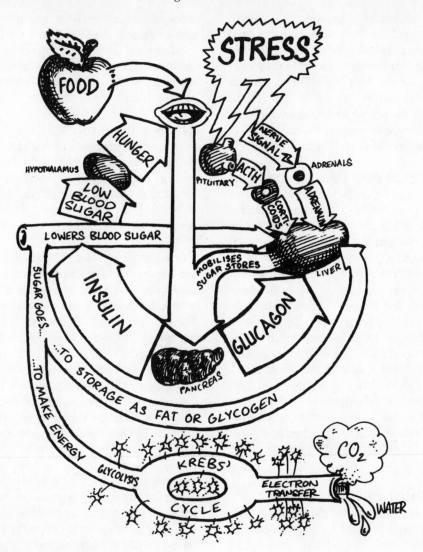

Figure 2.3.5 — *The sugar cycle*

The thyroid and metabolism

One of the long term effects of stress is to slow down the rate of metabolism. This inevitably leads to increasing difficulty losing weight. Your rate of metabolism can be likened to a fire. Those that have a fast rate of metabolism are 'fast burners'. They need constant stoking and are usually energetic and thin, or at least not overweight. Those with a slow metabolic rate are 'slow burners', and they need only the smallest amount of food to keep the fire burning. They usually have less energy and are overweight. The rate of metabolism is controlled by the thyroid gland, at the base of the throat. This gland produces a hormone, thyroxine, on stimulation from the anterior pituitary through its release of TSH. The pituitary stimulates metabolism as a response to exercise, a stress reaction, or on stimulation with, for example, coffee. It depresses metabolism when fasting or dieting to conserve body stores of fat.

The production of thyroxine depends upon the presence of iodine. A lack of iodine induces an underactive thyroid, characterized by weight increases, a reduction in appetite, sluggish digestion, hence constipation, lethargy and apathy. Fortunately lack of iodine is rare. However iodine is generally only found in foods grown near or in the sea. Fish and seaweed, such as kelp, are rich sources. Salt is now iodized and even though less people are adding salt there has been no increase in iodine deficiency, possibly due to more availability of foods from all over the world.

Sometimes the thyroid glands become over-active. This can be, and often is, the result of a tumour or proliferation of thyroxine-producing cells. This results in the speeding up of the metabolic rate and hence brings on a drop in weight and increase in appetite, more rapid digestion and hence diarrhoea, increased heart rate and blood-pressure, muscular tremors, nervousness, and the person tends to become excitable and apprehensive. Conventional treatment involves giving radioactive iodine. The iodine concentrates in the thyroid and, being radioactive, destroys a part of the thyroid gland. One of the radioactive isotopes given off from nuclear disasters is radioactive iodine. As a precaution iodine is then given to saturate the thyroid's iodine receptor mechanisms, thus preventing the radioactive iodine from damaging the thyroid gland.

Maintaining calcium balance

Different cells in the thyroid gland also produce a hormone involved in the regulation of calcium levels in the body. Since calcium is needed to trigger impulses in nerve and muscle cells, as well as to provide rigidity to bones, the regulation of calcium levels in the blood, and hence available to cells, is of critical importance. This regulation is provided by two hormones: calcitonin from the thyroid, and parathormone (PTH) from the parathyroids, which are four tiny endocrine glands situated on the back of the thyroid gland.

Parathormone raises blood levels of calcium. It does this by stimulating the mobilization of calcium from the bone; by increasing the re-absorption of calcium from the kidneys; and by converting vitamin D into a hormone which increases gut absorption of calcium. When calcium levels are too high the thyroid releases calcitonin which suppresses mobilization of calcium from bone.

The sex hormones

In the male the release of gonadotrophin from the anterior pituitary stimulates the testes to produce testosterone. This hormone stimulates the sexual characteristics of an adult male, including body and facial hair, voice changes, development of sex organs and increased sex drive.

In the female gonadotrophic hormones stimulate the ovaries to produce oestrogen and progesterone, which are responsible for female sexual characteristics and the menstrual cycle. The gonadotrophic hormone follicle stimulating hormone (FSH) starts the menstrual cycle by stimulating the Graafian follicles within the ovary to release oestrogen. Oestrogen effectively prepares the female sexual system for a potential conception. The stimulation of the Graafian follicles leads to the release of an ovum some fourteen days into the cycle, known as ovulation. At this point the corpus luteum within the ovary produces progesterone, while oestrogen release continues, although at an ever decreasing rate. These two hormones continue to prepare the female sexual system for possible conception, until their levels are sufficiently reduced to bring on menstruation. Menstruation is caused by the breakdown of the endometrium, the lining of the womb, to give menstrual flow.

In pregnancy the ovum is fertilized by a sperm and this encourages the corpus luteum in the ovary to continue growing and producing progesterone until it grows to occupy as much as 50% of the ovary. The increased level of progesterone maintains the pregnancy. By about the fourth month of pregnancy the corpus luteum becomes inactive and the placenta produces progesterone to maintain the pregnancy.

PART THREE

FOOD AND NUTRITION

CHAPTER 3.1

The macronutrients: protein, fat and carbohydrate

—OVERVIEW—

Of the thirty-eight different substances known to be essential for life, three are needed in relatively large amounts. These are proteins, fats and carbohydrates — the macronutrients.

Carbohydrates are our primary source of energy. Plants produce carbohydrates by combining carbon and oxygen, from carbon dioxide, with oxygen and hydrogen, from water. The energy needed for the plant to do this job is supplied by the sun. The process is called photosynthesis. Foods high in carbohydrates are fruits, vegetables, grains, and pulses. These should make up the majority of our diet providing at least 55% of our calories. In reality, the average diet is only 35% carbohydrate. But it isn't just a question of quantity. Quality is also important. Carbohydrates can be digestible or indigestible. the indigestible part is called fibre. The digestible part is further divided into complex or simple carbohydrate. Sugar is a simple carbohydrate, while beans provide good complex carbohydrate (or starch), which promotes good health.

Fats are also important. Fat protects us from the cold, provides cushioning for our organs and bones, insulates nerve cells from one another, and is a component of every human cell. Fat can also be converted into a form that can be used to provide energy. Fats come from the animal and vegetable kingdom. Fats from vegetables are mainly unsaturated. Animal fat is mainly saturated. Certain kinds of unsaturated fats are particularly important because they make hormone-like substances in the body called prostaglandins, which are essential for life. These are called essential fatty acids. Fats should make up no more than 30% of our calorie intake. In reality the average diet is 42% calories from fat.

Protein is vital for life since all our cells are made out of protein. Bone, hair, skin, nails are all different kinds of proteins. Proteins consist of amino acids. There are some 22 key amino acids which, depending on their arrangement, make up different proteins. Eight of these amino acids are called essential amino acids, because we must get them from our diet. The rest can be made by the body. A food that has all these amino acids is said to provide good quality protein. If the food has a high percentage of calories from protein then it is a good protein source. We get protein from the animal and vegetable kingdom. Grains, beans, lentils, nuts, seeds and sprouting seeds are all good protein sources. So are eggs, milk, cheese, meat and fish. Vegetarian sources of protein tend to be of poorer quality, and it is important that a vegan meal includes a mixture of plant proteins (e.g. cereals and pulses) so that they can make good each other's essential amino acid deficiencies. However animal protein sources tend to be too high in fat. Many of us get ample protein, providing over 20% of calories. We only need about 10-15% of our calories to come from protein.

—UNDERSTANDING CARBOHYDRATES—

Not all forms of sugar are bad for you. Sugar, our most important energy supply, comes in many different shapes and disguises, some of which are better than others. Sugar is a carbohydrate (made from carbon, hydrogen and oxygen). The more complex a carbohydrate is the longer it takes to digest into a simple carbohydrate, e.g. glucose, ready for absorption. Lentils, for example, are high in complex carbohydrate, while fruit contains a simple fruit sugar, fructose, and is therefore digested quickly.

Why complex carbohydrates mean more stamina

Foods containing complex carbohydrates therefore release their sugar load gradually over a longer period of time. This slow release makes them a better source for stamina and continued good energy. However, if you cook carbohydrate for too long it makes it easier for the digestive enzymes to get at the starch more quickly, which results in too much sugar being released too soon into the blood-stream. This sudden rise in blood sugar, often followed by a sudden drop, can cause all sorts of symptoms of discomfort ranging from sleepiness, mental confusion, irritability, depression, to dizziness, headaches and thirst. These result from the brain, the most glucose-dependent organ in the body, being flooded or starved of vital fuel.

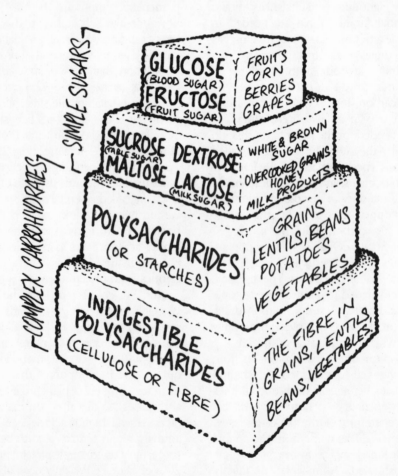

Figure 3.1.1 — *The sugar family tree*

Why fruit is better than sugar

Even though all carbohydrates ultimately end up as simply sugars, not all sugars have the same effect on one's blood sugar level. Besides glucose and fructose food sugars are of three types known as di-saccharides: maltose, sucrose and lactose. 'Di' means two, so these sugars are themselves a combination of two 'mono-saccharides', the choice being glucose, fructose and galactose. These three are the potential end products of sugar digestion. Glucose is the fastest releasing sugar and makes the blood sugar level shoot up most rapidly. Fructose, found predominantly in fruit is the next fastest, with galactose, from milk, lagging somewhat behind. So foods which ultimately end up as glucose are potentially worse for you than foods that end up as fructose or galactose.

Maltose, for example malt extract, is made up of two glucose molecules, so that's no better for you than straight glucose, as found in some fizzy 'high-energy' drinks. What we know as sugar is sucrose, made from one glucose and one fructose molecule, so that's marginally better, but not as good as straight fruit sugar. Milk sugar is made from a galactose and a glucose molecule and is therefore the slowest releasing of them all.

The effect that different tyes of sugar have on your blood sugar level can be measured. When sugar enters the bloodstream blood glucose levels rise. At a certain point the pancreas releases insulin (and the liver releases glucose tolerance factor) which helps to transport the glucose from the blood into the cells. This results in a decrease in blood sugar level. This change in blood sugar level can be plotted against time to give a blood sugar curve.

The space under the curve represents the degree of reaction a particular food has on the blood sugar level. As a standard, the curve created by pure glucose represents a score of 100 and the relation between the test food and the glucose effects is called the Glycaemic Index. In the chart below Dr Jenkins and Dr Wolever analysed many different foods to see what their effect on blood sugar was.

Grains had a small effect on blood sugar level, but when grains were refined the effect became

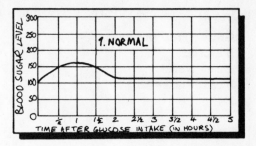

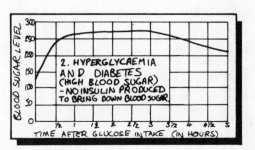

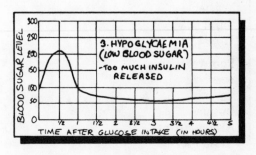

Figure 3.1.2 — *Blood sugar curve*

greater. Rice went from 66 to 72 when refined. The best grains in this test were buckwheat and wholewheat spaghetti. Of the breakfast cereals tested, cornflakes came out worst and porridge oats the best by a long way. Oat cakes also have little effect on blood sugar. Many root vegetables, particularly carrots and potato had a suprisingly large effect on blood sugar. This effect may be very dependent on the degree of cooking.

The Glycaemic Index of Common Foods

Grain, cereal products		Swede	72
Buckwheat	51	Yam	51
Bread (white)	69		
Bread (wholemeal)	72	**Pulses**	
Millet	71	Beans (tinned, baked)	40
Pastry	59	Beans (butter)	36
Rice (brown)	66	Beans (haricot)	31
Rice (white)	72	Beans (kidney)	29
Spaghetti (wholemeal)	42	Beans (soya)	15
Spaghetti (white)	50	Beans (tinned, soya)	14
Sweetcorn	59	Peas (blackeye)	33
		Peas (chick)	36
Breakfast cereals		Peanuts	13
All-bran	52	Lentils	29
Cornflakes	80		
Muesli	66	**Fruit**	
Porridge oats	49	Apples (golden delicious)	39
Shredded wheat	67	Banana	62
Weetabix	75	Oranges	40
		Orange juice	46
Biscuits		Raisins	64
Digestive	59		
Oatmeal	54	**Sugars**	
Rich tea	55	Fructose	20
Ryvita	69	Glucose	100
		Maltose	105
Vegetables		Sucrose	59
Broad beans	79	Honey	87
Frozen peas	51	Mars Bars	68
		Lucozade	95
Root vegetables			
Beetroot	64	**Dairy products**	
Carrots	92	Ice cream	36
Parsnips	97	Milk (skim)	32
Potato (instant)	80	Milk (whole)	34
Potato (new)	70	Yogurt	36

Chart 3.1.1 — *Glycaemic Index of Foods*[1]

The best foods from all those tested were pulses — peas, beans and lentils. None of these had a substantial effect on blood sugar. Milk products which contain the sugar lactose, were also good. Suprisingly, even ice cream came out well. But don't kid yourself — it's still high in fat and sugar, even if it doesn't alter blood sugar level much.

Fruits, being high in glucose as well as fruit sugar, had quite a strong effect on blood sugar.

Raisins, being concentrated, were the worst with bananas a close second. Apples were the best. But fruit sugar, fructose, had much less of an effect than glucose or maltose. Sucrose, which is table sugar, is a combination of glucose and fructose and was in between these two for its glycaemic rating. Very high up in the list were Lucozade, Mars Bars and even honey. Despite some interesting findings the overall effect is clear. Any form of concentrated sugar affects blood sugar balance.

Beans are particularly good because they contain 'polyphenols' which slow down the absorption of sugars. Their soluble fibre content also slows down glucose absorption. Beans are also naturally high in minerals. Fruit is naturally high in vitamins, particularly vitamin C. Both vitamins and minerals are needed to process the sugar once inside your body, so although not actually affecting your blood sugar immediately, sweet foods high in nutrients are considered more healthy.

Which forms of sugar are best?

Any food containing complex carbohydrate, or naturally rich in fructose and vitamins or minerals, is far better than refined sugar, honey or malt. That means beans, lentils, seeds, and grains and vegetables, as long as they're not over-cooked, as well as fresh fruit. Provided you avoid all forms of refined sugar, and don't have too much concentrated natural sugar as in pure juice (dilute it) or dried fruit, there's no reason to be concerned about how much sugar your diet provides.

If you do add sugar to food or drinks, or eat foods with sugar already added start using less or switch to fruit instead. The taste for sweetness will gradually decrease as your body gets used to more complex carbohydrates.

The importance of fibre

Although not a nutrient, indigestible forms of carbohydrate called fibre play a crucial role in the digestive system. Fibre was originally thought only to speed up the passage of digested food through the gastrointestinal tract thereby preventing constipation and putrefaction of food. However it is now known that some forms of fibre slow down the absorption of sugars and thereby help prevent high levels of sugars in the blood-stream. One of the most interesting types of fibre is a substance called glucomannan, from the Japanese Konjac plant. This fibre has been shown to have excellent weight-reducing properties and also helps to reduce insulin requirements for diabetics.

But not all forms of fibre are carbohydrate. Lignin, found predominantly in raw vegetables, is indigestible and helps to speed up gastrointestinal transit time.

A lack of fibre is associated with the increased incidence of many diseases of the colon, including constipation, diverticulitis, colitis, irritable bowel syndrome, colon and rectal cancer. The average person in Britain consumes 20g of fibre a day, compared to the average British vegetarian, who consumes 42g per day. During the war intake of dietary fibre was somewhere between 32-40g on average. Africans living in rural communities consume between 50 and 120g per day. There is strong evidence that an intake of at least 30g per day is associated with a lower incidence of these diseases of the bowel, and thus the NACNE (National Advisory Committee on Nutrition Education) report recommended this level as a minimum guideline.

—FACTS ON FAT—

Are you sitting comfortably? If so, it's because of fat. Contrary to popular opinion fat is actually good for you. It keeps you warm, is a store of energy, keeps your skin and arteries supple, protects you from heart disease and allergies and balances your hormones. It's even essential for proper brain function, which is, incidentally, one-third fat. But just how much and what kind of fat you eat makes all the difference. The NACNE report recommends us to get no more than 30% of all our calories from fat, while the average intake is more like 42%. But perhaps more important than this is the kind of fat you eat.

Saturated fat

Saturated fats (which are generally solid at room temperature) are only really useful as a source of energy and padding. But since most of us eat enough calories to give us energy and have a little too much padding, you don't really need them. If you're running out of fat, the body's long-term store of energy, provided you're eating enough carbohydrate foods like grains, beans, lentils or fruits, you can convert these into saturated fat. The highest sources of saturated fats are meat produce, cheese, eggs and fast food, which often includes fat simply because it's a cheap ingredient and makes you feel full fast. Meats like pork and beef are the worst, with up to 80% of their calories coming from fat. But even eggs, which have a reputation for being a good source of protein, are 66% fat. Cheese varies from 74% (cheddar) down to 19% (cottage cheese). New low fat cheeses have about half as much fat as normal cheese. Other foods that are high in fact include avocados (82%), coconut (80%) and some nuts and seeds, although these are pre-dominantly unsaturated.

There is no danger in eating some saturated fat. It is good fuel. But there is a danger in eating too much. Strokes, heart attacks, breast cancer, diabetes, gallstones and acne are some of the diseases associated with a high saturated fat intake.

Butter or margarine?

Unsaturated fats can be turned into saturated fats by a process called 'hydrogenation'. This is used in margarine manufacture to render the vegetable oil solid at room temperature. This process also changes the nature of unsaturated fats from the natural 'cis' form to 'trans' fatty acids, losing the qualities of polyunsaturated fats. Hydrogenated unsaturated fats are no better for you than saturated fats, the major component of butter. Some of the better margarines have unprocessed unsaturated oils added back which are of some benefit.

Essential fatty acids

While unsaturated fats can be used for everything that saturated fat is used for, some unsaturated fats have a special role to play in making hormone-like chemicals that control many body functions, as well as being incorporated into every cell in our bodies. There are called 'essential fatty

acids' or EFAs and are the topic of chapter 3.4.

Cholesterol

Another fat essential for health is cholesterol. It is a normal component of the body tissues, especially those of the brain, nervous system, liver and blood. It acts as a lubricant for the arteries, and is needed to make adrenal and sex hormones, as well as vitamin D and bile, which helps in the digestion of fats.

Since gallstones and deposits found on the artery walls in arteriosclerosis contain cholesterol it has been theorized that they are the result of high cholesterol diets. But there is considerable evidence to show that the dietary intake of cholesterol makes only a small contribution to the body levels of cholesterol. It has been suggested that the cholesterol may even effect a 'puncture repair'. However the building up of cholesterol, fats and calcium, presents a later danger of arterial blockage. Excess dietary cholesterol would therefore be a contributive factor, but not the cause.

Lecithin

One fat which helps to break down fats is lecithin. It may act as a 'washing-up liquid' to break down other fats into tiny particles that can be carried through the walls of the arteries and out of the blood. Bile, the digestive secretion from the gallbladder, contains lecithin which breaks down fats into smaller units which the pancreas enzyme lipase can then work on.

Interestingly enough eggs, which are a high source of cholesterol, also contain plenty of lecithin. But when we interfere with nature by frying the egg, the lecithin is destroyed while the cholesterol remains. By eating them boiled or baked the initial balance is maintained.

Lecithin is also found in soya beans and corn, supplements usually being extracted from soyabeans. Apart from its emulsifying effect on fats, it is an important constituent of the brain, nervous system and adrenals.

—UNDERSTANDING PROTEIN—

Protein means 'of prime importance'. Seventeen per cent of our total body mass is protein. Protein actually consists of carbon, hydrogen, oxygen and nitrogen, often sulphur and sometimes phosphorus. For example cystine and methionine are sulphur-containing amino acids.

Protein has various functions. First of all it is used in structural roles in bones, skin, hair and muscle. Secondly protein is used for various substances in the body which cause specific effects; such as enzymes which help to change a substance from one form into another. For example, amylases, the carbohydrate digesting enzymes, are made of protein. Hormones and neurotransmitters (which are substances which which cause transmission of nerve signals) are often made of or from protein or amino acids. Insulin, the hormone that controls blood sugar, is a protein and the neurotransmitter serotonin, which helps you to fall asleep at night, is made from the amino acid tryptophan.

The structure of protein

Protein consists of long chains of amino acids. These amino acids are the building blocks of protein. When two amino acids combine it is called a peptide. If many combine the structure is called a polypeptide. When this structure becomes very complex it is called a protein. The combination of two or more amino acids gives rise to a peptide plus the by-product water. Now when we digest proteins down to peptides, and from peptides down to individual amino acids, the reverse process occurs. By the chemical combination of water with protein, which is done by the enzymes proteases, the separate amino acids are released. This is called hydrolysis, which means splitting with water.

Both in the liver and in individual cells these amino acids are then combined to make thousands of different kinds of proteins in a complex process involving RNA and DNA.

The essential amino acids

During the course of evolution, mankind lost the ability to make some amino acids so they must be supplied from diet. These are the essential amino acids. Though not essential in the diet because the body can make them itself, the other amino acids have essential roles in the body. The 'non-essential' amino acids are those present in body proteins but which do not have to be present in the food. — alanine, aspartic acid, cysteine and cystine, glutamic acid, glycine, hydroxyproline, proline, serine and tyrosine. Other amino acids with important functions in the body but which are not present in the body proteins include: taurine, carnitine, GABA and ornithine. Another semi-essential amino acid is histidine which is essential in childhood but considered non-essential in adulthood. However, we do need some dietary sources of histidine which in turn gives rise to histamine, a very important chemical in the body.

—THE AMINO ACIDS—

Essential	Semi-essential	Non-essential and therapeutic
Leucine	Arginine	Proline
Lysine	Histidine	Taurine
Isoleucine		Carnitine
Threonine		Tyrosine
Tryptophan		Glutamic acid and Glutamine
Methionine		Cysteine and Cystine
Valine		Glycine
Phenylalanine		Alanine
		GABA
		Ornithine

Chart 3.1.2 — *The key amino acids*

The third type is amino acids which are produced from other amino acids and as such may have a role in protein synthesis, but they can be extremely useful for other reasons. An example is tyrosine, present in dietary protein and made from the essential amino acid phenylalanine. Tyrosine is involved in the production of the hormone adrenalin. Since a low level of tyrosine can induce depression and physical lethargy it is not surprising to find that supplements of tyrosine can help relieve depression. See Leon Chaitow's book *Amino Acids in Therapy* for more details (Thorsons, 1985).

Complete protein

Leaving the therapeutic uses of amino acids till later, the primary need to eat protein is to make body protein. A food which contains the eight essential amino acids in approximately the right proportions is called a complete protein. The highest sources of complete protein are eggs, fish, meat, milk, cheese and yogurt. These foods eaten on their own provide us with usable protein. However it is a mistake to think of these as our only sources of complete protein.

Complementary proteins

If one food has a deficiency in two amino acids and it is then combined with a food that is strong in these two amino acids the result is a complete protein. For example, rice is deficient in isoleucine and lysine but sufficient in the sulphur amino acids, while broad beans are strong in the amino acids isoleucine and lycine but low in the

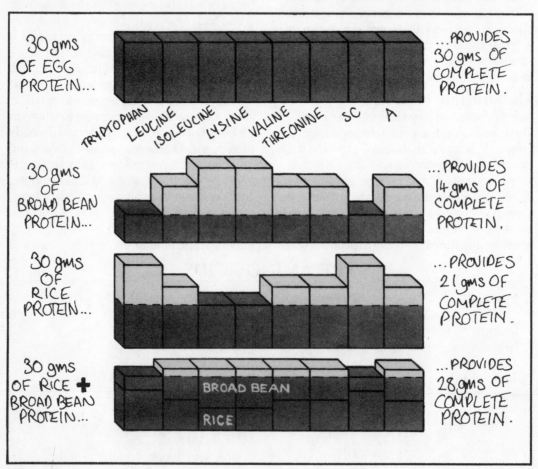

Figure 3.1.3 — *Making a complete protein*

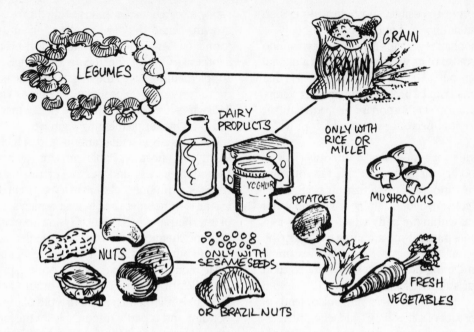

Figure 3.1.4 — *Combining foods for more complete protein*

sulphur amino acids. These foods combined are therefore a good source of plenty of complete protein without eating any meat, fish, eggs or milk products.

Since the body does have a pool of amino acids in circulation which is filled both from diet and also from the breakdown of body proteins it is not necessary that all these complementary foods are eaten at the same meal.

Amino acids in therapy

There are to date around 142 documented diseases which occur due to errors in metabolism. Many of these errors are in protein metabolism. Some are acquired often due to poor nutrition or exposure to anti-nutrients such as chemicals, pesticides or heavy metals. In some disease states it is necessary to supplement amino acids to achieve optimal help. In other circumstances it is wise to know how one can obtain these amino acids from diet.

Glycine is a non-essential amino acid which the body can make. During times of rapid growth such as childhood, very large amounts of glycine are needed. It is also needed to make haemo-

globin which helps transport oxygen around the body. Glycine is also important for the production of DNA as well as helping to eliminate certain toxins from the liver.

Glutamic acid is used in the formation of several non-essential amino acids. In a purified form it's used as a flavour enhancer as in monosodium glutamate, used in Chinese foods. Glutamic acid is also important in the synthesis of a neurotransmitter called GABA. GABA is considered to be a primary inhibitory neurotransmitter in the brain preventing nerve cells from discharging a nerve impulse. L-glutamine, yet another relative of glutamic acid, has been shown in animals to reduce the craving for alcohol.

Phenylalanine and tyrosine, which can be produced from phenylalanine, are used in the production of adrenalin and also the thyroid hormone called thyroxine as well as the skin pigment melanin. In Addison's Disease the adrenal glands fail to make enough adrenalin. This leads to the diversion of phenylalanine and tyrosine to make more melanin resulting in a deepening skin pigmentation. While the body can convert phenylalanine into tyrosine the reverse is not possible, so phenyalanine is an essential amino acid and tyrosine is not.

Tryptophan is perhaps the best known amino acid because of its widespread use as a natural sleeping pill. The reason for this is that tryptophan can be broken down into serotonin. Serotonin is a very important neurotransmitter in the central nervous system which provides sleep.

Histidine is an essential amino acid in childhood as the body is unable to synthesize sufficient amounts during that time. Histidine can be converted to histamine, a very powerful chemical within the body which also acts as a neurotransmitter. If you are stung by a wasp the itchiness and swelling are caused by a histamine reaction. During the hay fever season, the reaction to pollen is also a histamine reaction. People who produce too much histamine also tend to produce a lot of saliva, have headaches, allergies and a variety of other symptoms. Some people genetically produce too little histamine, and histidine — its precursor — can be an important constituent of diet although it is not in fact a totally essential amino acid.

Ornithine can be produced from arginine which at the moment is showing some inter-esting research results and is being dubbed the growth factor due to its effect on muscle formation. Arginine is also needed in protein synthesis. One of the theoretical dangers of supplementing large amounts of arginine is for those carrying or exposed to the herpes virus. This virus lives off arginine and hence may be activated by supplementing arginine.

Lysine is an essential amino acid which is lacking in most vegetable proteins with the exception of peas and beans. For this reason lysine is commonly deficient in a vegetarian diet. Lysine is sometimes used to treat certain strains of the herpes virus.[2] Since lysine resembles arginine chemically the virus takes up the lysine instead but cannot flourish and hence dies off.[3]

Methionine, cysteine and cystine are all examples of sulphur-containing amino acids. Sulphur is important for certain types of protein bonding and is partly responsible for the formation of keratin in hair. Sulphur has a role in the structure of the very important hormone insulin which controls our blood sugar level. Sulphur-containing amino acids also help to detoxify certain heavy metals and encourage the absorption of selenium. Good dietary sources of sulphur include onions, garlic and eggs.

CHAPTER 3.2

The micronutrients: vitamins

—OVERVIEW—

The macronutrients are required directly for energy production and tissue repair. However they could not function without vitamins. Just about every chemical reaction that takes place within the body is regulated by a special enzyme and many enzymes are dependent on vitamins, notably the B vitamins. Enzymes are the key to human biochemistry and hence to optimum health, and vitamins are the key to optimum enzyme function.

Many vitamins have an associated deficiency disease that results from an overt deficiency of the vitamin or mineral in question. For instance scurvy results from vitamin C deficiency, and rickets from vitamin D. Much of the early research into vitamins and minerals went into discovering the levels of each vitamin required to prevent its associated deficiency disease. From these levels a safety factor was added on and the resulting figure was declared the RDA (recommended daily amount) for the nutrient.

But does just preventing deficiency disease ensure optimum function? The overwhelming result of more recent research is 'no, it certainly doesn't'. And due to current practices of refining and processing many foods causing substantial losses of nutrients, many people are getting far from optimum levels of these nutrients. Indeed marginal deficiencies of vitamins and minerals are probably the most common cause of sub-optimum health.

A vitamin is a chemical compound that cannot be synthesized by the human body. All vitamins are originally manufactured in the green leaves of plants and are then transferred to the seed of the plant to nourish the next generation. We obtain vitamins either by eating the plant directly or through eating animals which have previously eaten plants and stored the vitamins. Vitamins A, D and E are fat soluble and can be stored in the body while vitamins B and C are water soluble and must be replaced on a daily basis. The key to a vitamin is its chemical structure, and this can be broken down by exposure to heat or light. Thus fresh foods have the highest vitamin content.

—VITAMINS—

The word vitamin denotes a substance that is essential for life. Any substance whose deficiency would result in death, illness or impairment in normal body processes, such as growth, that cannot be made by the body is classified as a vitamin (unless it is a mineral, essential amino acid or essential fatty acid). However there are other substances that we can make but not in large enough amounts to ensure optimum health. An example of a semi-essential nutrient is choline.

The discovery of vitamins began at the turn of the century, at a time when medical science was mainly concerned with drugs or antidotes to illnesses. So when it was discovered that vitamin C within lemons prevented scurvy in 1932, it came to be understood that vitamin C was the anti-scurvy factor. Later on we discovered B_1 to be the anti-beri-beri factor and in the mid-thirties discovered B_3 to be the anti-pellagra factor. In each of these instances, a number of defective signs developed before the overt deficiency disease appeared. For example, it takes 200 days deprivation of vitamin C before scurvy develops, however during this time resistance to infection decreases, as does energy and mental concentration.

It is increasingly realized that RDAs which are intended to satisfy the requirements of most people *in a group*, have often been misinterpreted and used as the requirement *for an individual*. Any one individual may need more than the RDA of one nutrient and less than the RDA of another, and these requirements may alter with the changes in the way of life or physiological state. This earlier notion that deficiency of a vitamin would cause a specific disease is a distortion of our present understanding of how vitamins work. We are, if you like, hairy bags of salty soup with many chemicals interacting through the action of enzymes and these make up how we feel and how we function. Since these enzymes are interactive, any imbalance in one can cause an imbalance in another. However, it was not until the 'fifties that some researchers began to realize the interactive quality of nutrients. The appreciation of this synergy between vitamins, and their ability to affect health even when not acutely deficient, has begun to change nutrition from a static science into a dynamic one.

—FAT SOLUBLE VITAMINS—

Vitamin A

The fat soluble vitamins are vitamins A, D, E and K. A comes mainly through two sources. One is retinol — the animal form of vitamin A, which comes from organ meats, dairy products, eggs and fish and therefore tends to be well supplied in a more carnivorous diet. The other form is beta-carotene. Beta carotene isn't strictly vitamin A. It's called provitamin A because it's a precursor of vitamin A. The intestines can convert six units of beta-carotene into one unit of retinol. In fact this figure is a little arbitrary because the more beta-carotene you take the less is converted into retinol. Also, if liver stores are high less beta-carotene is converted. This mechanism is probably a natural safeguard against toxicity for our ancestors who obtained most of thier vitamin A from vegetables. Both forms of vitamin A are measured in ius or international units. Generally speaking 1.98mcg of beta-carotene equals 1iu,

while 0.33mcg of retinol equals 1iu.

What does it do?

Vitamin A strengthens the skin, both inside and out, and also the lungs and gastrointestinal tract against infection. It is also essential for making a pigment in the eyes called rhodopsin which is needed for black and white vision. The release of vitamin A from liver stores is dependent on zinc, and people might show symptoms of vitamin A deficiency but in fact be zinc deficient. Beta-carotene in its own right has recently been shown to have a role as an anti-oxidant which can function in areas of low oxygen tension, for example cancer cells. It is high in raw vegetable juices which may explain why these have been effective in helping cancer patients.

Toxicity

The optimum daily intake is anything between 20 and 30,000iu rather than the recommended daily allowance of 2,500iu. However, it is the most toxic of all the vitamins and megadoses should not be taken without professional advice. Certain synthetic derivatives of vitamin A, called 13 cis-retinoic acid, used primarily for people with acne and serious skin disorders have been shown to be toxic in doses less than 50,000iu. Since these synthetic compounds have been shown in animal studies to be teratogenic (which literally means 'monster producing' in terms of birth defects) it would be advisable for a pregnant woman not to take in excess of 10,000iu of any form of vitamin A. However, in the form of beta-carotene it does not appear to be quite so toxic.

Vitamin D

Vitamin D is only found in foods of animal origin, the best sources being in fish, liver, eggs and liver oils, vitamin D is also added to milk in some countries such as the USA. Deficiency is much rarer since most of our vitamin D is synthesized in the skin. However dark skinned people filter out the harmful ultra violet rays, a natural adaptation to living in a warm climate, and this also prevents the production of vitamin D in the skin. Vitamin D deficiency is therefore more likely to occur in Asian and African immigrants who come to this country and remain well clad most of the time. Vegetarians are also more at risk from deficiency.

What does it do?

Vitamin D is needed for the absorption of calcium and therefore the primary sign of deficiency is rickets in children and osteomolacia in adults, where the bones literally become bendy due to a lack of calcium. Other signs are muscle cramps, osteoarthritis, joint aches and pains. The recommended intake is between 400 and 1,000iu. Children need proportionately more.

Vitamin E

Vitamin E is called tocopherol, derived from the Greek word for childbirth for the reason that wheatgerm oil which is rich in tocopherols is said to increase fertility in animals. Vitamin E is found in nuts, seeds and vegetable oils which it helps to prevent from becoming rancid. One unnamed company in America removes the vitamin E from vegetable oils and sells it to vitamin companies who manufacture it. So you should ensure all vegetable oils are cold-pressed or raw (untreated).

The active form of vitamin E is called d-alpha tocopherol. Some supplements contain mixed tocopherols which, weight for weight, are far less potent. Others contain the synthetic d-alpha tocopherol which is about 36% less potent than the same weight of the natural form.

What does it do?

Vitamin E is an anti-oxidant, protecting fats within the body from oxidation. It is thought to aid the transport of oxygen so is good for people with poor circulation, atherosclerosis or thrombosis. It is therefore absolutely vital for people suffering from arterial disease. However, vitamin E can make the heart muscle very effective and if the arteries are blocked it can cause palpitations. This can be avoided by using not more than 200iu and building the dose up gradually to a maximum of 1,000iu a day. Its anti-oxidant properties may be useful in protecting against cancer. Vitamin E also makes a good moisturizer and the application of vitamin E cream helps to heal wounds. Deficiency induces infertility in animals however there is no substantial evidence that taking vitamin E will increase fertility in humans. There is good evidence for general supplementation of 100/200iu of vitamin E per day although doses of up to 1,000iu may be needed for people with special needs.

Vitamin K

Vitamin K is not supplemented to any great extent because it can be produced by bacteria in the gut. It is involved in blood clotting and really only ever presents a problem in young infants. There is a particular factor in breast milk which prevents the uptake of vitamin K by the infant if the mother is very deficient. Cauliflower and cabbage are particularly high in vitamin K so it is important for nursing mothers to eat these.

All the fat soluble vitamins can be stored in the body and therefore do not need to be supplied religiously on a daily basis.

—THE WATER SOLUBLE VITAMINS—

The water soluble vitamins are divided into vitamin C and the B complex group of vitamins. The B complex includes B_1 (thiamine), B_2 (riboflavine), B_3 (niacin), B_5 (pantothenic acid), B_6 (pyridoxine), B_{12} (cyanocobalamine), folic acid and biotin. Also sometimes included are choline and inositol, which although they can be synthesized by the body and hence are not strictly vitamins, they act much like vitamins in the body and are semi-essential in that dietary intake is of significance as some people do not synthesize adequate quantities of these substances.

Vitamin C

Vitamin C is unlike any other vitamin in that we can tolerate and may function better on levels of this vitamin that far exceed the Recommended Daily Amount. While the average intake is in the region of 40mg a day (an orange provides up to 60mg) most people can absorb 2,500mg a day and estimates of optimal intake have ranged between 1,000 and 10,000mg a day. Green peppers, oranges and kiwi fruit are rich sources of vitamin C, however most fresh fruit and vegetables will contain some.

It is likely that we, like all other animals except guinea pigs, fruit bats and apes, used to make vitamin C. In most animals it is synthesized from glucose and it is thought that we may have lost the ability to make vitamin C at sometime during our evolution. In a tropical environment rich in dietary sources of vitamin C, this would have been advantageous since more glucose would have been available for energy and less for providing vitamin C, allowing greater mobility and less reliance on frequent eating. However if the climate then changed as it did in the ice age this inability to produce vitamin C would become a disadvantage. Animals that do produce it will produce an equivalent amount of about 3,000mg a day and under stress this may go up to 10,000mg.

Another theory used to explain our great need for vitamin C revolves around histamine. Histamine is one of the neurotransmitters in the body which is in part responsible for speeding up oxidation reactions which generate body heat. Being a natural anti-histamine, producing large quantities of vitamin C would depress the histamine level and therefore depress body temperature. So it may be to our advantage not to produce it and get it from dietary sources.

What does it do?

Vitamin C strengthens the immune system and encourages productions of lymphocytes which fight infection. Vitamin C is also required during the syntheses of collagen which is our intercellular glue. It is a powerful anti-oxidant and protects the body from carbon monoxide in a polluted environment or generated from cigarette smoke. It has been shown that blood vitamin C levels are lower in smokers. Vitamin C also helps to remove lead from the body and prevents the formation of a carcinogen (cancer producing substance) called a nitrosamine, which can form in the stomach from the combination of nitrites and amines when vitamin C levels are low.

The Bioflavonoids

Vitamin C is found in nature with a group of substances called the bioflavonoids (which used to be called vitamin P). These include rutin, which strengthens capillaries and polyphenols which influence blood sugar and fat levels. As these compounds may potentiate the effects of vitamin C they are often taken in conjunction with vitamin C.

B_1 — Thiamine

B_1 is needed for carbohydrate metabolism and may become deficient in those on a high sugar diet. It is vital for maintaining the integrity of the nervous system, and helps make the neurotransmitter acetylcholine. Prolonged deficiency results in neuritis, oedema, and psychological disturbance among other symptoms collectively known as beri-beri. Beri-beri is extremely rare, however it may occur with people whose diets are very high in sugar or alcohol. There is some evidence of marginal B_1 deficiency being associated with low levels of intelligence in school children.

B$_2$ — Riboflavin

B$_2$ is an orange/yellow coloured vitamin. High or excessive intake may discolour urine. However, since B$_2$ is not toxic this is perfectly safe. Because of its strong colour it is sometimes used as a safe food additive. Symptoms of deficiency include overacidity, sore tongue, oily hair, eczema and cataracts (these can be improved with supplementation).

B$_3$ — Nicotinic acid

B$_3$ comes in two forms: nicotinic acid and nicotinamide. In America these are called niacin and niacinamide. Both forms act as the vitamin, however the niacin or nicotinic acid form also acts as a vasodilator causing a release of histamine. This effect can easily be experienced by taking 100mg of niacin. This causes a blushing sensation and change in temperature as perhiperal circulation improves. The vasodilatory effect helps take nutrients to cells and remove toxins and also changes the stickiness of the blood. It is often effective in stopping migraines and headaches. Niacin has also been shown to be effective in treating some schizophrenics.

B$_5$ — Pantothenic acid

B$_5$ is found in nearly every food, hence its name derived from Greek, pantos, meaning every-where. It is vital for making the neurotransmitter acetylcholine and is thought to boost memory. It is also needed by the adrenal glands to make the glucocorticoids which may be the reason that it's called an anti-stress vitamin, and has been found to be helpful in arthritis. It is non-toxic and can be used in relatively large amounts.

B$_6$ — Pyridoxine

Since B$_6$ was shown to be effective in preventing pre-menstrual tension, it has attracted bad publicity with regards to toxicity. This may have occurred because B$_6$ is not designed to be taken in isolation, but should be taken with other B vitamins and the mineral zinc. The best nutritional results for the treatment of pre-menstrual syndrome lie with the supplementation of B$_6$, zinc and magnesium together with dietary changes. B$_6$ has been shown to be toxic in doses of 2,000mg upwards . A symptom of toxicity is peripheral neuropathy, experienced as tingling in the extremeties. This is most unlikely to occur in doses much below 200mg.

Vitamin B$_{12}$

B$_{12}$ is called cyanocobalamine and is known as the anti-pernicious anaemia factor. It is the only vitamin that contains a mineral, cobalt, hence its name. To be used by the body it requires the presence of 'intrinsic factor' produced in the stomach. It is essential for the production of red blood cells which carry oxygen, and is also needed to make DNA which is the blueprint for all cells. B$_{12}$ helps make the myelin sheath that insulates nerves. Symptoms of deficiency include anaemia, smooth and sore tongue, tremors, lassitude, menstrual problems, mental disorders. B$_{12}$ is found in all animal produce such as meat, eggs, milk and is scarce in the vegetable kingdom. It is found in comfrey and also in large amounts in spirulina, which is a form of algae. Vegetarians are advised to take a supplement since little is supplied through the diet. The major problem with pernicious anaemia is one of absorption and therefore pernicious anaemia is treated by injection. B$_{12}$ is supplied as cyanocobalamine in supplements. Only 1% of dietary intake is absorbed. There is no evidence that extra cobalt intake affects B$_{12}$ status. A small amount of calcium is needed for absorption.

Folic acid

As with B$_{12}$, anaemia will result when folic acid is low. Amounts of folic acid in supplements are restricted since it can mask B$_{12}$ deficiency by curing anaemia, although the nerve degeneration characteristic of B$_{12}$ deficiency still carries on. Deficiency may be associated with an increased risk of spina bifida, a neural tube defect in babies of folic acid deficient mothers. It is needed to make RNA and DNA and is therefore essential for the manufacture and repair of all cells. It also helps to regulate histamine levels in the body. Deficiency signs include anaemia, weakness, fatigue, breathlessness and mental symptoms. Much more is needed during pregnancy, especially for those who have previously had a miscarriage. As a sensible precaution against the possibility of masking a B_{12} deficiency, folic acid should not be taken without a basic intake of B_{12}. However, this does not help if there is a lack of intrinsic factor.

Biotin

Biotin is a rather ignored B vitamin which was discovered when raw egg white consumption resulted in illness. Avidin, a protein in egg which is destroyed by cooking, induces biotin deficiency. Biotin is involved in the metabolism of proteins, fats and carbohydrates. It helps maintain healthy skin, hair and a balanced hormonal system. The symptoms of deficiency, anaemia, dermatitis, scaly skin and diarrhoea, are rare but do sometimes occur in babies. It is also needed to make delta-6-desaturase, an enzyme that converts essential fatty acids into precursors of their respective prostaglandins. Biotin can be synthesized in the intestine when the right bacteria are present.

PABA

PABA stands for para-amino-benzoic-acid (which is why it is abbreviated). It is needed for healthy skin and hair growth, with a particular function in skin pigmentation. It is a very effective sunscreen applied to the skin and is used to treat vitiligo, a condition in which the parts of the skin lose their colour. Prevents grey hair in some animals. It has not been established as essential in man.

Choline

Choline is a constituent of lecithin and can be made by the body so strictly speaking it is not a vitamin. It helps make acetylcholine and is therefore essential for brain function. In large amounts choline may improve memory and mental function. As a constituent of lecithin it helps to break down accumulating fats in the liver. Signs of circulatory disease, such as high blood-pressure or excess cholesterol may be partly due to choline deficiency. Choline can be taken in the form of choline bitartrate or phosphatidyl choline (lecithin). Choline chloride has the unfortunate side effect of leaving you smelling like dead fish.

Inositol

Inositol is also a constituent of lecithin and again is not strictly a vitamin since it can be made by the body. Its function isn't known, however it is found in large quantities in the nerves. Inositol can be taken in lecithin or by itself. It is usually within a B complex tablet. Used in doses of 1,000mg a day it is said to have a mild tranquil-lizing effect, however this has not been confirmed by all researchers.

CHAPTER 3.3

The micronutrients: minerals

—OVERVIEW—

More than a hundred years ago a Russian chemist called Mendelyeff noticed that all the basic constituents of matter, the elements, could be arranged in a pattern according to their chemical properties. From this he produced the Periodic Table. There were many gaps where elements should be, and sure enough over the years these missing elements have been discovered. All matter is made out of these elements.

Some of these are gases, like oxygen and hydrogen, some are liquids such as mercury and some are solids such as iron, zinc and chromium. We are mainly made up of carbon, hydrogen and nitrogen, as well as minerals which make up 6.1% of our body weight. The minerals that are known to be essential for life are mainly used to regulate and balance our body chemistry, with the exception of calcium, phosphorus and mag-

nesium which are the major constituents of bone. These minerals are required in tiny amounts compared to carbon, hydrogen and oxygen. For instance, a 10-stone man needs 400 grams of carbohydrate a day and .015 grams of zinc. Yet zinc is no less important.

Minerals are originally extracted from the soil by plants. Like vitamins, they may be obtained directly from plants or indirectly via meat. Unlike the vitamins the chemical structure of minerals is not so critical and they can be absorbed and utilized by the body in a variety of different forms. But since many recently discovered minerals remain unrecognized both by health departments and the food industry these are frequently refined out of foods as there is no legislation yet to replace them. Therefore they are more likely to be deficient in man.

—THE MACRO-MINERALS—

Those minerals that are present in the body in relatively large amounts are known as the macro-minerals. These include calcium, magnesium, phosphorus, potassium, sodium and possibly iron.

Calcium
Nearly 3lbs of your body weight is calcium and 99% of this is in your bones and teeth. Calcium

is needed to provide the rigid structure of the skeleton. Its need is particularly high in childhood when bones are growing and also in the elderly because the ability to absorb calcium becomes impaired with age. The remaining 10 or so grams of calcium are in the nerves, muscles and the blood. It is needed for nerve muscle cell activity and that which is in the blood is either in the process of transportation or helps the blood to

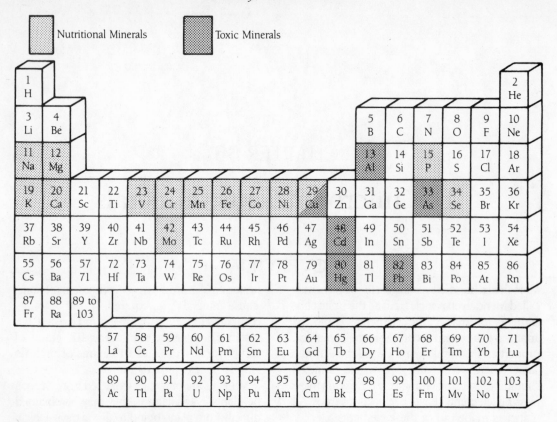

Figure 3.3.1 — *The periodic table*

clot and help maintain the right acid/alkaline balance.

The average diet provides marginally less than the RDA for calcium, with most of this coming from milk and cheese. However vegetables, pulses, nuts, wholegrains and water provide significant quantities of calcium too.

The ability to use calcium depends not only on its intake but also its absorption. Normally only 20 to 30% of calcium is absorbed. Absorption is increased by exercise and adequate vitamin D status, and a greater proportion is absorbed when dietary intake is low. It is made worse by a deficiency of vitamin D, exposure to lead, consumption of alcohol, coffee and tea or a lack of hydrochloric acid. The presence of phytate, excessive phosphorous or fat in the diet also intereferes with absorption. Once in the body calcium availability is lessened by excessive protein consumption.

Symptoms of deficiency include muscle cramps, tremors or spasms, insomnia, nervousness, joint pain, osteoarthritis, tooth decay and high blood-pressure. Severe deficiency causes osteoporosis, or porous bones. This makes them fragile and prone to fracture. Osteoporosis is particularly prevalent in post-menopausal women, since the lack of oestrogen also negatively affects calcium absorption. It is now known that even a supplement of 2,000mg daily only slightly slows the rate of bone loss after the menopause, yet 73% of women get less than 500mg a day.

Magnesium

Magnesium works together with calcium both in maintaining bone density and in nerves and muscles. The average diet is relatively high in calcium but deficient in magnesium, because milk is our major source of calcium and is not a very good source of magnesium. Both calcium and magnesium are present in green leafy vegetables, nuts and seeds. It is a vital component of chlorophyll which gives plants their green colour and therefore is present in all green vegetables. However, only a small proportion of the magnesium within plants is in the form of chlorophyll.

Magnesium is involved as a co-factor in many enzymes in the body, working together with B_1 and B_6. It is also involved in protein synthesis and hence a co-factor in some hormones. It may be its role in hormone production or prostaglandin production that is responsible for its beneficial effects in treating pre-menstrual problems. But its most important role is its balance with calcium in maintaining proper nerve and muscle impulses.

A lack of magnesium is strongly associated with cardiovascular disease in that individuals dying from coronary heart disease have abnormally low levels of magnesium in the heart. A lack of magnesium causes muscles to go into spasm and there is considerable evidence that some heart attacks are caused not by an obstruction of the coronary arteries but by cramping of the arteries leading to oxygen deprivation of the heart.

Sodium

Sodium is eaten mainly in the form of sodium chloride (salt). Of the 92g of sodium in the body more than half is in the fluids surrounding cells where it plays a vital role both in nerve transmission and the maintenance of normal water concentration in blood and body fluids. Deficiency is exceedingly rare both because it is added to foods in excess and also because its excretion is under careful homeostatic control by the kidneys. It is present in most natural foods in small amounts and is mainly supplied in processed foods.

An excess of sodium is associated with a raised blood-pressure although it appears that some people are not salt-sensitive in this way. As sodium levels in the body rise fluids are made less concentrated by retaining more water. This gives rise to oedema or fluid retention.

Potassium

Potassium works in conjunction with sodium in maintaining water balance and proper nerve and muscle impulses. Most of the potassium in the body is inside the cell. The more sodium is eaten the more potassium is required, and since the average intake is 6 grams of sodium and up to 3 grams of potassium relative deficiency of potassium is widespread. An equivalent intake of these two is more consistent with good health. Fruits, vegetables and wholegrains are rich in potassium.

Severe potassium deficiency may result in vomiting, abdominal bloating, muscular weakness and loss of appetite. Potassium deficiency is more likely to occur in those taking diuretic drugs, laxatives, or long-term use of corticosteroid drugs.

Iron

Iron as the red pigment, haem, is a vital component of haemoglobin which transports oxygen and carbon dioxide to and from cells. Sixty per cent of the iron within us is in the form of haem iron. This is the form present in meat and it is much more readily absorbed than the non-haem iron present in non-meat food sources. Non-haem iron occurs in the oxidized or ferric state in food, and not until it is reduced to the ferrous state (for example by vitamin C) during digestion, can non-haem iron be absorbed.

THE BIOAVAILABILITY OF IRON	
	% Available
Steak	95
Corned beef	95
Bran	75
White bread	57
Boiled egg	10

Chart 3.3.1

The symptoms of iron deficiency include pale skin, sore tongue, fatigue or listlessness, loss of appetite and nausea. Anaemia is clinically diagnosed by checking haemoglobin levels in the blood. However symptoms of anaemia can be caused by a lack of vitamin B_{12}, folic acid, and also be deficiency of vitamins C, E and B$_6$ and copper. Iron deficiency amaemia is more likely to occur in women, especially during pregnancy. Since iron is also an antagonist to zinc, supplements containing more than 30mg of iron, over twice the RDA, should not be given without ensuring adequate zinc status. Although often supplemented in doses above 50mg there is little evidence that this is more effective in raising haemoglobin levels than lower doses. Folic acid, now often also given as a supplement to pregnant women, also appears to be an antagonist to zinc.

—THE TRACE ELEMENTS—

Zinc

A large part of the population is at risk of being zinc deficient. Neither hair nor blood tests show zinc deficiency accurately. The zinc taste test appears quite good but has not yet undergone rigorous testing. This test involves tasting a weak solution of zinc sulphate. If you cannot taste this then zinc deficiency is suspected. The solution is available in some health food shops. Deficiency symptoms are white marks on the nails, lack of appetite, pallor, acne, impaired fertility, lack of resistance to infection, mental and emotional imbalance. Zinc deficiency is mentioned as a factor in nearly every major disease, i.e. diabetes and glucose intolerance. Zinc is needed to make insulin and to boost the immune system and make the anti-oxidant enzyme SOD. Zinc is required to make prostaglandins, which are hormone-like substances, from essential fatty acids. These are important in maintaining the right stickiness of the blood so may be a factor in treating heart disease. Sucking zinc lozenges may be at least as effective as taking vitamin C in cutting short a cold. Zinc's main role is the protection and repair of DNA and for this reason zinc is highest in animals who have high levels of DNA. So the vegetarian diet may be low in zinc. Stress, smoking and alcohol deplete zinc and also sex since semen has a high concentration of zinc. Oysters are popularly said to be aphrodisiacs. They are also the highest dietary source of zinc and for both the male and female zinc is essential for fertility.

Manganese

Manganese is known to be involved in no less than twenty enzyme systems in the body. One of the most critical is one of the SODs (superoxide dismutase) which acts as an anti-oxidant, helping to disarm free radicals. In animals manganese deficiency also results in a lowered production of insulin. Since diabetics frequently have low manganese status it is thought to be involved in maintaining blood sugar balance. It is also involved in the formation of mucopolysaccharides, a constituent of cartilage. One of the first signs associated with deficiency is joint pain.

Manganese is also required for proper brain function. Deficiency has been associated with schizophrenia, Parkinson's disease and epilepsy. It is frequently deficient in the diet and best sources include tropical fruits, nuts, seeds and whole grains. Tea is also a significant source of this mineral and supplies half our daily intake. Little more than 5% of manganese eaten in the diet is absorbed and there is evidence that supplemental manganese is also very poorly absorbed.

Copper

Copper is both a nutritional and a toxic element. It is required in man in doses as little as 2mg a day. It is rarely deficient for the simple reason that most water supplies are contaminated with copper from copper pipes. Some say it is deficient particularly in those with a high zinc intake. It is needed in the formation of the insulation myelin sheath around nerves and is also a constituent of one of the SOD anti-oxidant enzymes. Copper and zinc are strongly antagonistic and a deficiency in zinc may lead to a greater absorption of copper. Likewise, excessive zinc supplementation can induce copper deficiency.

It is wrongly included in multimineral tablets and used in many cooking utensils. The birth control pill also increases copper levels. All these factors make it relatively easy to accumulate too much copper, which is associated with schizophrenia, cardiovascular disease and possibly rheumatoid arthritis. However, a deficiency of copper has also been associated with rheumatoid arthritis. Copper is involved in an anti-oxidant enzyme involved in some inflammatory reactions. This may be the reason why too much or too little can result in greater inflammation in those with rheumatoid arthritis. Copper levels rise during pregnancy and it is speculated that it plays a role in bringing on labour.

Chromium

Chromium is a vital constituent of glucose tolerance factor, a compound produced in the liver which is thought to help transport glucose from the blood to the cells. Vitamin B_3 and the amino acids glycine, glutamic acids and cystine are also required for glucose tolerance factor. Continued stress or frequent sugar consumption therefore deplete the body of chromium. A diet high in refined foods is also likely to be deficient in this mineral since it is found in wholegrains, pulses, nuts, seeds and especially in mushrooms and asparagus. Chromium supplements have been used successfully in the treatment of diabetes and glucose intolerance (see Chapter 4.5).

Selenium

Selenium deficiency was first discovered to lead to a specific disease in China, where a type of heart disease called Keshan disease was discovered in areas in which the soil was deficient in selenium. It has since been discovered to be a factor in another regional disease, this time in Russia, involving joint degeneration. Perhaps the most significant finding in relation to selenium is its association with a low risk of certain kinds of cancer.

Selenium is the vital constituent of the anti-oxidant enzyme, glutathione peroxidase. A tenfold increase in dietary selenium causes a doubling of this enzyme in the body, illustrating the enzyme's dependence on selenium. Since many oxides are cancer-producing and since cancer cells destroy other cells by releasing oxides, it is likely to be selenium's role in glutathione perioxidase that gives it protective properties against cancer and premature ageing.

Selenium is found predominantly in wholemeal flour and in seafoods and seeds, especially sesame seeds.

The micronutrients: essential fatty acids

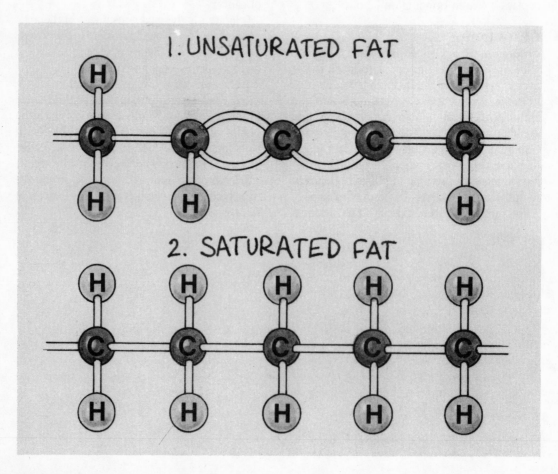

Figure 3.4.1 — *Saturated vs unsaturated fat*

Contrary to popular opinion some fat in the diet is actually good for you. It keeps you warm, is a store of energy, keeps your skin and arteries supple, protects you from heart disease and allergies and balances your hormones. It's even essential for proper function of the brain, which is, incidentally, one-third fat. But just how much and what kind of fat you eat makes all the difference. The NACNE report recommended us to get no more than 30% of all our calories from fat, while the average intake is more like 42%. But more important than this is the kind of fat you eat.

While unsaturated fats can be used for everything that satured fat is used for, some unsaturated fats have a special role to play in making hormone-like chemicals that control many body functions, as well as being incorporated into every cell in our bodies. These are called 'essential fatty acids' or EFAs. To understand why they are so vital for health requires some understanding of their structure.

Imagine you have in front of you a load of ping pong balls, some marked C for carbon, and others H for hydrogen, and some rods. The balls can be attached to the rods in four places. Now all fats contain fatty acids which consist of a chain of these carbon atoms. But saturated fatty acids have each hole above and below filled, or satured, with hydrogen. Unsaturated fatty acids have one or more 'double bonds' where the holes are not filled. If it's got one double bond it's oleic acid, found in olive oil, if it's got two double bonds it's called linoleic acid, and if it's got three double bonds it's called linolenic acid, high in seed oils. Unlike saturated fatty acids they are liquid at room temperature and are found predominantly in the vegetable kingdom and especially in nuts and seeds. Fish is also high in unsaturated fatty acids. After all, consider what would happen if a fish was high in saturated fat and entered cold water — it would solidify!

The essential fatty acids

Linoleic acid and linolenic acid are essential for life itself. You could think of them as vitamins. Linoleic acid derivatives make hormone-like substances called prostaglandin series 1 and 2, which are involved in inflammatory reactions and also in the stickiness of the blood. If you lack lineoleic acid the result can be eczema, allergies, pre-menstrual tension and even

hyperactivity. An alpha-linolenic acid derivative makes prostaglandin series 3, this time involved in keeping the heart and arteries healthy, again influencing the formation of blood clots.

Evening primrose oil helps eczema

When we eat these fats the body gradually makes the fatty acid more and more complex by adding on extra carbon atoms and double bonds. As shown below, linoleic acid has an extra double bond added and turns into gamma-linolenic acid (GLA), of which one of the highest known sources is the evening primrose plant. Borage seeds and blackcurrant seeds are even richer sources.

Because evening primrose oil contains GLA, which is one step nearer to being a prostaglandin, research has found it to be an effective treatment for eczema, asthma, pre-menstrual tension (PMT) and hyperactivity. But since it is also expensive

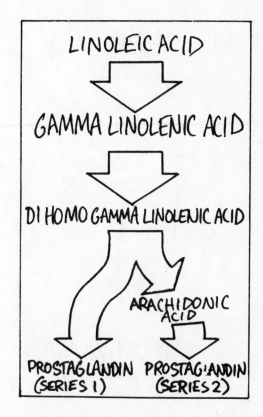

Figure 3.4.2 — *Diagram of linoleic acid pathway*

why not just eat more vegetable oils, rich in lino-leic acid? The problem is that not everybody is very good at coverting linoleic acid into gamma linolenic acid. This conversion depends on an enzyme, delta-6-desaturase, which is dependent on vitamin B_6, biotin, zinc and magnesium. So if you're deficienct in these nutrients, or if you drink too much or are under stress the ability to convert becomes further impaired. Some PMT sufferers get more benefit by supplementing B_6 and zinc, for example, and eating more cold-pressed oils, while others respond best to evening primrose oil.

Alpha-linolenic acid, may also be difficult to convert into prostaglandins because the conver-sion also depends on the enzyme, delta-6-desaturase. However, fish oils contain a derivative of alpha-linolenic acid called eicosapentaenoic acid (EPA) from which Series 3 prostaglandins are made.

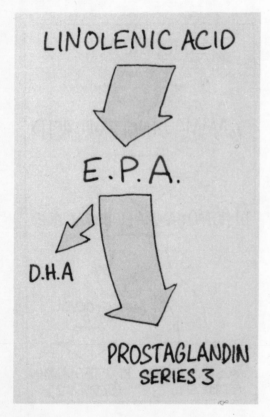

Figure 3.4.3 — *Diagram of alpha-linolenic acid pathway*

This prostaglandin series 3 helps protect our heart and arteries in many ways. It reduces blood levels of two fats associated with heart disease, cholesterol and triglycerides. It thins the blood, thus minimizing the risk of blood clots that lead to heart attacks and strokes. Even so, research using high concentrations of EPA has shown much stronger effects on promoting healthy arteries than just eating more vegetable oils. Unfortunately, the only natural source of EPA is fish that have in turn eaten the plankton rich in alpha-linolenic acid. It's this special oil that has protected the Eskimos from heart disease despite eating a high cholesterol and high fat diet.

But not everything about these unsaturated fats are good for you. One other semi-essential fatty acid called 'arachidonic acid' encourages inflam-matory reactions. Although we need to have some to make the series 2 prostaglandins, too much can mean a greater risk of eczema, asthma and allergies. Meat and milk are the highest sources of arachidonic acid. No wonder many asthma and eczema sufferers find milk aggravates their condition and a vegetarian diet helps it. Anyway we can make arachidonic and hence the series 2 prostaglandins from linoleic acid, even though much more of the anti-inflamma-tory series 1 prostaglandins are made, which would appear to be the right balance for health.

Vegetarian diets reduce cancer risk

This mainly appears to be because their total fat intake is low. For many years it has been known that vegan diets, without any meat, fish, eggs or dairy produce, and plenty of vegetable juices can have remarkable healing power for cancer patients. Many theories have been evoked to explain why, but a recent discovery points to essential fatty acids being the answer. Cancer cells, being generally rather inefficient, have great difficulty converting the linoleic acid into arachidonic acid. This makes them dependent on dietary sources of arachidonic acid. But a vegan diet starves them of this and provisional laboratory experiments suggest that cancer growths diminish rapidly with this selective malnourishment.

But, according to American statistics, people eating a diet too high in these polyunsaturates actually have a higher risk of cancer. How could this be? As well as being essential for making prostaglandins, these complex polyunsaturated fats are very vulnerable to damage. Their many double bonds leave them open to attack by dangerous peroxides. These peroxides, called free radicals, can set up a chain reaction of damage making the oil go rancid. Peroxides are particularly present in unsaturated oils when heated, and a diet too high in vegetable fats, containing a lot of fried food could well mean more free radicals. Once inside the body free radicals will home in on double bonds. These are either found in unsaturated fats incorporated into cell walls, or in DNA, the very genetic code of the cell. If either get damaged the cell might become wrongly programmed and turn cancerous.

Warning: Don't cook with vegetable oils

Nature is well aware of this weakness and provides adequate vitamin E, an anti-oxidant, in foods rich in unsaturated oils. But some food manufacturers actually take out the vitamin E from vegetable oils and sell this dismembered oil to an unsuspecting public, and, in turn, sell the vitamin E to the vitamin manufacturers! It is for these reasons that it is best to buy cold-pressed (or raw) untreated vegetable oils and to keep them in the fridge to minimize oxidation. The same applies to a lesser extent with nuts and seeds. These are packed with essential oils. Nuts and seeds should always be bought fresh and eaten quite quickly. Nuts that are split to be shelled, like walnuts, are more prone to oxidation than almonds, for example. These precautions are not so essential with olive oil since it is only a monounsaturated fat and has only one double bond. (This is why it goes solid if refrigerated.) Because polyunsaturated fats are prone to oxidation when heated it is best not to fry with

these but to use a small amount of butter or olive oil. Butter, being mainly saturated fat has no double bonds, and olive oil being monounsaturated, only has one, and subsequently less chance of creating free radicals. But either way, frying should be avoided as much as possible.

Which is better: butter or margarine?

As well as being prone to oxidation some kinds of food processing can make polyunsaturated fats lose their ability to make prostaglandins. When margarine is made unsaturated fats are 'hardened' by a process called hydrogenation. By adding in hydrogen to the double-bonds the fat becomes more saturated. So when you see on a food label 'hydrogenated vegetable oil' read 'saturated fat' because that's effectively what you're getting. Some margarines have a greater degree of polyunsaturated oils added back. Vitaquell contains the highest amount of unhydrogenated polyunsaturated oil. In the case of margarines like Flora and Vitaquell, they are made mainly from non-hydrogenated vegetable oils plus smaller amounts of hydrogenated vegetable oils. By law no food can claim to be 'polyunsaturated' unless at least 45% of its fatty acids are polyunsaturated in the naturals cis : cis form and less than 25% are saturated. 49% of the fatty acids in butter are saturated and only 2.24% polyunsaturated. Use butter or margarine for spreads as little as possible. Alternatives are diluted tahini, or nut spreads which don't need butter as well.

In summary we all need some polyunsaturated fat but not a lot. The equivalent of two table-spoons of polyunsaturated oils is ample each day. That could be a handful of nuts or seeds, or a dressing on a salad. To preserve essential fatty acids avoid frying as much as possible and bake or grill instead. If you do fry, use butter or olive oil for as short a time as possible. For other purposes use cold-pressed vegetable oils kept in the fridge.

CHAPTER 3.5

Balancing your diet

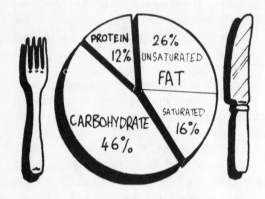

COMPOSITION OF AN AVERAGE DIET

Figure 3.5.1 — *The average diet*

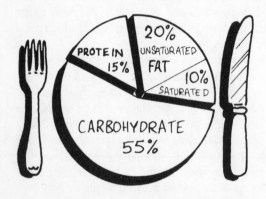

COMPOSITION OF AN OPTIMUM DIET

Figure 3.5.2 — *The optimum diet*

Although many of us like to think we eat a well balanced diet surveys have shown that few people actually know what a well balanced diet is. Most people eat too much fat and not enough complex carbohydrates. Sugar and fat are both high in calories per ounce; while one cup of fat and sugar provides 2,500 calories, you'd need a whole bucket of fruit and vegetables to get the same amout.

The NACNE report, commissioned to provide dietary guidelines for a healthier nation, recommends eating no more than 30% of calories from fat, 11% from protein, and 50% from carbohydrate, assuming 5% will come from alcohol. They also advise that not more than one-third of the fat should be saturated. Polyunsaturated fats provide the essential fatty acids. Of the carbohydrate foods, they advise that the refined sugar consumption per person per year should be cut from 84lbs (38kg) to 75lbs (34kg). British school children at present eat 79lbs a year, on average.[5]

In practical terms you should decrease your fat intake, eat fish rather than meat, and then only three times a week. Experiment with vegetarian forms of protein like beans, lentils and grains. Boil or bake instead of frying and switch to skimmed milk. Cut down on cheese and choose cottage cheese or Edam which are lower in fat. Avoid sugar, instead use fresh and dried fruit to sweeten food. Most of all make fresh fruit and vegetables a substantial part of your diet.

Balancing your vitamins and minerals

Even many people who think they are eating a well-balanced diet may not be getting all the recommended levels of vitamins and minerals. A mainly vegetarian diet, high in raw fruit and vegetables will score high on most B vitamins and trace elements, and provides as much as 40,000iu of vitamin A. But it is often lacking in B_{12}, B_6, vitamin D and zinc. On the other hand, a diet high in meat and without so much whole foods is likely to lack some of the B vitamins and the rarer trace elements like manganese, chromium and magnesium which are predominantly found in plant foods.

If you're thinking that you can't win you're right, at least as far as vitamins and minerals are concerned. It's almost impossible to eat a diet that provides enough of all these nutrients for the optimum health regime advocated in this workbook. And every dietary survey conducted in Britain in the last eight years has come to the same conclusion. The NACNE report concluded that '10% of the population get less than 30 mgs of vitamin C a day' (RDA is 45mg). The Bateman report said '85% of the women and their families ate a diet which did not provide the daily nutrient intake recommended by the DHSS'[4] The 1986 Booker Report found even more alarming evidence shown in the table below.[6] That's why most nutritionists recommend nutritional supplements on top of a good diet to ensure optimum nutrition.

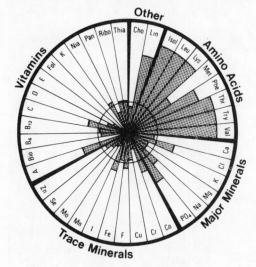

Figure 3.5.3 — *The average diet*

Nutrient	% of men below RDA	% of women below RDA
Vitamin C	93	95
Folic acid	93	98
Calcium	—	73
Iron	60	—
Zinc	—	57

Chart 3.5.1 — *Results of Booker Health Survey 1986*

Below we've tried our best to design the best possible all round diet to give you an idea of what level of nutrition you can get from food.

— BANANA BREAKFAST —
A delicious combination of natural yogurt, banana, wheatgerm, crunchy coconut, dates and sunflower seeds.

— RAINBOW ROOT SALAD —
A colourful combination of raw grated carrots, beetroots and parsnips with an island dressing made from tomatoes, tofu manyonnaise, carrot and almond meal.

— SPAGHETTI NAPOLITANA —
Wholemeal spaghetti with a sauce of carrots,

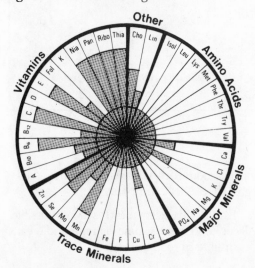

Figure 3.5.4 — *The optimum diet*

tomatoes and mushrooms, flavoured with thyme. Serves with a generous sprinkling of parmesan cheese and watercress salad.

— RASPBERRY SORBET —
Frozen raspberries and bananas liquidized to a smooth purée.

As snacks throughout the day — three pieces of fruit in season, including an apple eaten with a piece of cheddar cheese. Drink Barley cup, dandelion coffee, red zinger, lemon mist or any other Celestial Seasoning herb tea.

What this diet provides for an average 2500 calories per day.
FAT:24% (Polyunsaturates — 75%, saturates — 25%)
PROTEIN:10%
CARBOHYDRATE:66%

Vitamins:	What this diet provides	RDA*	Optimum*
A	— 35,000iu	2,250iu	7,500
D	— 50iu	100	400
E	— 15iu	—	400
C	— 159mg	30	2,000
B_1	— 1.2mg	1.2	25
B_2	— 1.5mg	1.6	25
B_3	— 12mg	18	50
B_5	— 4.5mg	—	50
B_6	— 2.9mg	2	50
B_{12}	—1.2mcg	3	10
Folic acid	264mcg	300	300
MINERALS			
Calcium	— 750mg	500	800
Magnesium	— 400mg	400	400
Potassium	— 4,3000mg	—	4,000
Sodium	— 434mg	2,000	1,000
Zinc	— 7mg	11	15
Iron	— 11mg	12	12

*RDA — where there are no British RDAs, US RDAs or World Health guidelines have been used instead.

*Optimum levels calculated from research at Institute of Nutrition.

Chart 3.5.2 — *A well balanced diet*

To help you balance your diet here are 11 basic principles to follow.

1. Make sure at least half your diet consists of alkaline-forming foods which are all vegetables, fruits, sprouted seeds, yogurt, almonds, brazils, buckwheat.

2. The rest of your diet should consist of acid-forming foods such as grains, pulses, nuts, seeds, eggs, cheese, fish and poultry.

3. Eat all food (except meat) as raw as possible. All cooking destroys some vitamins and breaks down fibre in food.

4. When using oils other than for cooking (salad dressings, spreads, mayonnaise) use cold-

pressed sunflower, sesame or safflower oils.

5. Drink at least half a pint of water a day between meals. For other drinks try diluted fruit juices and herb teas.

6. Avoid foods with added salt. Don't add salt to your cooking or your food. It isn't needed.

7. Avoid sugar and other foods with concentrated sweetness. Honey and maple syrup are only marginally better. Dilute fruit juice and soak dried fruit.

8. Avoid fatty meats like beef, pork and lamb and other high fat foods. Have more vegetarian sources of protein.

9. Avoid processed and 'fast' foods with long lists of additives or preservatives.

10. Avoid frying foods. Grill or bake instead. If you do fry use olive oil or a small amount of butter for as short a time as possible.

11. Avoid regular consumption of tea or coffee. On average, don't drink more than a glass of wine, spirit or pint of beer a day.

Special diets

Different diets have been associated with different countries, and even different religions and philosophies throughout the world. Among those that have become most associated with health are macrobiotics, vegetarians, veganism and food combining.

Macrobiotics

Macrobiotics is based on the principle that all of life can be viewed as a balance between two energies: yin and yang. These energies can be seen in all aspects of life including nutrition. For example, woman is yin, man is yang. Night is yin, day is yang. All foods can also be classified as being degrees of yin or yang. However the degree of yin or yang is relative. For example fruit is considered yin. But with fruits apples are the most yang. These energies attract each other and by balancing yin and yang in all aspects of life health and well-being is achieved. The following foods are classified as yin, yang or in-between within their food groups.

YANG	IN-BETWEEN	YIN	YANG	IN-BETWEEN	YIN
A general guide			Pumpkin	Cabbage	Tomato
Animal food	Cereals	Dairy produce	Garlic	Lentil	Aubergine
Eggs	Vegetables	Fruits	Radish	Celery	
Fish	Nuts	Sugar	**Dairy foods**		
Meat and fish			Goat cheese	Milk	Cream
Pheasant	Chicken	Pork	Goat milk	Cream cheese	Margarine
Eggs	Beef	Eel		Butter	Yogurt
Turkey	Sole	Clam	**Fruits**		
Salmon	Trout	Oyster	Apple	Olive	Fig
Sardine	Halibut		Strawberry	Almond	Banana
Herring	Muscle		Chestnut	Melon	Grapefruit
Shrimp	Lobster		Cherry	Orange	Pineapple
Cereals			**Drinks**		
Buckwheat	Millet	Rye	Chicory	Herb teas	Champagne
Rice	Oats	Corn		Water	Tea
Wheat	Barley			Wine	Coffee
Vegetables				Fruit juice	Sugared drinks
Dandelion	Onion	Green peas		Beer	
Watercress	Parsley	Mushroom	**Miscellaneous**		
Carrot	Lettuce	Spinach	Sesame oil	Olive oil	Honey
Turnip	Chick peas	Potato	Corn oil	Lard	
Leek	Cauliflower	Asparagus	Sunflower oil	Molasses	

Chart 3.6.1 — *Yin and Yang in foods*

From a conventional point of view a macrobiotic diet has many advantages in that it very much encourages the eating of unrefined foods and reduces the intake of stimulants and intoxicants. However it is not without its inconsistencies.

Firstly, in practice a macrobiotic diet often provides large amounts of salt in gomasio (a mixture of sesame seeds and salt), miso or shoyu (made from soya). Most food is also cooked and fresh fruit is limited because it is too yin. For this reason adequate intake of B and C vitamins is not always possible. The macrobiotic approach also shuns the use of nutritional supplements claiming that a truly balanced diet will provide all essential nutrients. While this viewpoint is shared in principle by many nutritionists the sad truth is that in today's polluted world it is often necessary to supplement vitamins and minerals to ensure adequate intake. (The macrobiotic diet is often unsuitable and inadequate for infants and young children.)

Vegetarianism

Over 1.5 million people in Britain are vegetarian, eating no meat and fish, and a further 1.5 million avoid all red meat. Vegetarianism is nothing new. Even the Greek mathematician Pythagoras was vegetarian. He reasoned, somewhat tangentially, that instead of offering animal sacrifices to the gods, he could offer his mathematical equations. And like his equations, he believed in keeping his diet and body in equilibrium. A recent survey by Dr Lockie and researchers at the University of Surrey has produced slightly different equations on the diets of vegans (eating no animal produce), ovo-lacto-vegetarians (eating dairy products and eggs), and wholefood omnivores (80% of the diet from vegetables, cereals and wholegrains) compared to the average omnivore.

Vegan diets came closest to matching the NACNE standards for a healthy diet. However their diets did confirm previously reported deficiencies in B_2, B_{12} and vitamin D. Ovo-lacto-vegetarians had too much fat in their diet. However, they did have low blood levels of cholesterol, thought to be due to high fibre intake, which can lower cholesterol levels. The wholefood omnivores still ate too much fat and

didn't get that much more fibre, while the average omnivores got too much fat and not enough folic acid. The researchers concluded:

Those people on a near vegan or vegetarian diet can more easily meet currently approved dietary goals. It may be prudent to restrict the intake of flesh foods to twice a week, which is the average intake in primitive tribes adopting the 'hunter-gatherer' lifestyle.

The protein myth

Animal produce is the primary source of protein in the typical western diet. But is it the best kind? To judge the best source of protein, two factors must be considered. Firstly, whether the food contains the right proportion of the essential and semi-essential amino acids, and secondly how much protein is supplied in each gram of food.

Egg protein, for example, provides the right mix of amino acids, making it 94% usable. Grains, on the other hand, lack the essential amino acids isoleucine and lysine which limit its usuability to around 60%. These amino acids are called the limiting amino acids. Eggs provide 14g of protein in 100g of egg, the rest being mainly fat of one sort or another. So 100g of egg provides 14g of protein of which 94% can be used.

Complementary proteins

Animal produce, gram for gram, is only a marginally better source of protein than nuts and seeds, and it is not better than soya beans or milk produce. It is also a better source of fat. By combining vegetable-origin foods, which complement each other's limiting amino acids, it isn't hard to get protein that is as good as meat in net usability. Only a few vegetable-origin foods have such a high percentage of protein, so one would naturally need to eat more beans and rice, for example, than steak, to get the same protein. But since beans and rice are high in complex carbohydrate and fibre, this is an asset not a liability. (Figure 3.1.4 in chapter 3.1 shows which food groups, when combined, provide more usable protein.)

Micronutrients and the vegetarian

Another popular myth about meat is that it is

the only source of many vitamins and minerals. Meat does tend to contain plenty of iron in an available form, and also more zinc and vitamin B_6. But a recent survey at the University of Carolina showed no sign of increased relative deficiency in these nutrients for vegetarians compared to meat eaters. While the bioavailability of iron in a steak is 95% compared with 10% for the iron in an egg, simply eating a meal high in vitamin C can increase iron absorption fivefold. A boiled egg and a glass of orange juice is a good combination.

Of greater concern for the vegetarian is the mineral zinc. This is poorly supplied in foods of vegetable origin and — depending on where the food is grown and whether phosphate fertilizers (which prevent zinc uptake) have been used — can be deficient in the vegan diet. Since the recommended daily intake is 15mg and the average daily intake in Britain is between 9mg and 10mg, it is not just vegetarians who need to be concerned. In the study at the University of Carolina 30% of the vegetarians and 22% of the non-vegetarians were found to have low zinc status. Vitamin B_6 is also found in larger amounts in animal produce because of its role in protein metabolism. Although cooking will destroy some of the B_6, it is likely that a vegetarian diet may be low in this too.

Fat soluble vitamins A, D and E are relatively high in animal produce because they can be stored. The levels will, of course, vary according to the nutrition of the animal in question. However, vitamin A is well supplied in leafy vegetables, and particularly carrots and beetroot, so provided these are often eaten the vegetarian need not fear. Vitamin D is made in the skin in the presence of sunshine. Vitamin E is highest in nuts and seeds.

The vitamin most associated with deficiency in the vegetarian diet is B_{12}. However, this is only a potential problem in vegans, as milk and eggs provide plenty of B_{12}. So do fermented soya products, spirulina, comfrey . . . and bugs. A survey on vegetarians in India identified bugs as a protective factor against B_{12} deficiency!

Do vegetarians live longer

Judging by the records to date it is unlikely that being completely vegetarian has major advantages for life extension, compared to those whose meat consumption is low. Izumi, aged 120, the oldest man in the world, easts small quantities of fish, and Anna Williams, aged 112, Britains oldest inhabitant, eats less meat than average. Our ancestral diet was one of plenty of foods from vegetable origin, together with infrequent consumption of fresh meat. We have evolved to thrive on such a diet, and can equally thrive on one without meat. Vegetarians are less likely to suffer from hypertension or obesity. However they have no better statistics for most types of cancer. Fewer vegetarians smoke compared to meat eaters, so these results may not be due to diet.

Veganism

A vegan diet is the same as a vegetarian diet except that no animal produce, including eggs and dairy produce, is eaten. This further restricts the sources of protein making the selection of protein rich foods, such as beans and lentils, and the combination of foods more crucial. A vegan diet is also far more likely to be deficient in vitamin B_{12}, D, calcium, iron and zinc since all of these are supplied in dairy produce and eggs (except for calcium which is not found in eggs to any appreciable extent).

The potential deficiency of calcium is easily overcome by eating sufficient green leafy vegetables, wholefoods, nuts, pulses and seeds. Also soya milk (a healthy alternative to milk) is quite a good source of calcium. Iron is quite well supplied in wholegrains, lentils and beans and becomes much more bioavailable if eaten in conjunction with vitamin C rich foods. B_{12} does come in some vegetarian foods. Spirulina, a blue-green algae available in supplement form is particularly rich. Vitamin D can be made in the skin in the presence of sunlight, but is otherwise hard to get and zinc is richest in wheatgerm and other nuts and seeds. So while it is generally prudent for a vegan to supplement these essential nutrients a carefully balanced vegan diet could be suffcient. This will depend on the individual's requirements, lifestyle, exposure to sunlight and other factors.

Food combining

In 1920 Dr Hay, one of the early pioneers of nutrition, proposed that the proper combination of foods would promote health and longevity. He reasoned that since carbohydrates are predominantly digested in the mouth and intestines in a more alkaline environment, needing little time in the stomach, and since proteins were mainly digested in the more acid environment of the stomach, then protein and carbohydrate-rich foods would be digested better if eaten separately. Of course, almost all foods contain a combination of protein and carbohydrate, however most foods are predominantly one or the other, with the exception of beans and lentils. These, he argued, were more prone to cause indigestion and flatulence because of their combination of protein and carbohydrate.[7]

In addition to the non-combination of protein-rich and carbohydrate-rich foods was the idea of eating fruit separately from other foods. Fruits and vegetables are said not to mix. The sugars and acids in fruits slow the digestion of the starches in vegetables and may cause fermentation, bloating or gas. Acid fruits are best eaten separately from sweet fruits, and melons, although an excellent food, are thought to be hard to digest and best eaten on their own.

The diagram below shows which foods can and cannot be combined according to the Hay diet.

As with many special dietary regimes the kinds of foods recommended are consistent with healthy eating but not all the explanations fit the facts. Firstly, it is known that the reason some beans and lentils cause indigestion or flatulence is the presence of trypsin (protein digesting enzymes) inhibitors, indigestible proteins and soluble fibres. Trypsin inhibitors are contained in chick peas, soy beans, kidney beans and broad beans. These are largely broken down by cooking or sprouting, and the presence of some indigestible proteins, although providing food for colonic bacteria which then produce gas, is hardly consistent with ill health. Also, in an organism as complex as the human body it is unlikely that evolution would not have developed some method for coping with the combination of foods. After all, not all animals eat only one food at a time.

However the fact remains that there is plenty of anecdotal evidence that particularly those with digestive problems do experience better health when combining foods according to the recommendations of Dr Hay.

Acid/alkaline balance

All food has an alkaline or acid effect on the body. An excess of acid is known to cause indigestion, rheumatic conditions, headaches, aching muscles, and general exhaustion. Recent research has shown that 'eating alkaline' not only relieves these problems but has a positive effect on health and vitality. According to nutritionist Celia Wright, eating alkaline leads to a sense of 'overwhelming well-being, calmness, emotional stability and a feeling of constant optimism'. It also decreases the craving for cigarettes, alcohol and sugar.[8] Criminologist, Dr Alex Schauss has reported that all addictions actually decrease on an alkaline diet.[9] This was vividly illustrated by a study at New York's Columbia University which showed that smokers put on an alkaline diet found it much easier to give up.

All the foods we eat are processed, or metabolized, by the body. Depending on the components present in the food a residue is left which has a net alkaline or acid effect. It's a bit like burning a food and measuring the ash. Foods high in calcium, magnesium, sodium or potassium tend to more alkaline-forming, while those high in nitrogen, phosphorus, sulphur or chlorine are more acid-forming. A typical Western diet is up to 80% acid-forming including acid foods like meat, eggs, bread, cereals and cheese. Tea and coffee and any alcoholic drink also adds to the acid burden. The body is balanced 80% alkaline 20% acid. Ideally your diet should also be 80% alkaline containing large quantities of fruits, vegetables, seeds and some nuts. Even fruits like oranges are alkaline-forming. Although their immediate effect in the stomach is one of acidity because of its chief

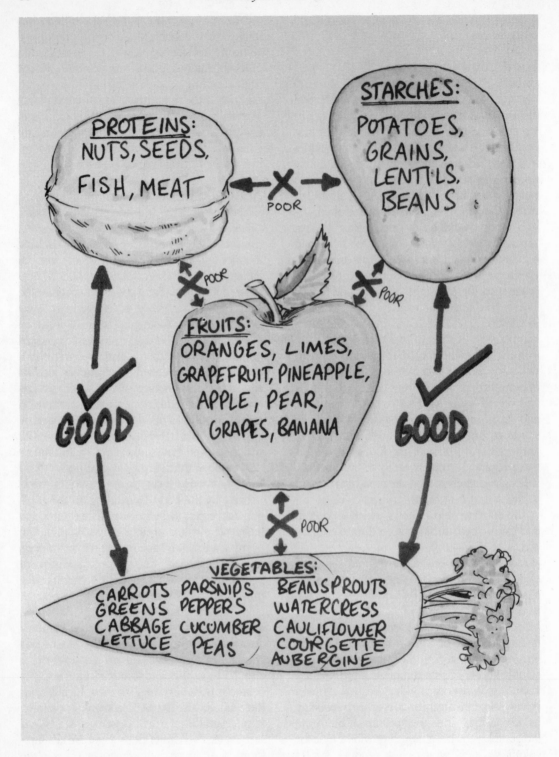

Figure 3.6.1 — *Food combining*

ingredient, citric acid, once digested all fruits are alkaline and highly beneficial.

Eating an acid/alkaline balanced diet has more benefits besides. It's naturally high in vitamins, minerals and fibre, and low in sugar and fat. In fact it's the ideal recipe for vitality and just what our ancestors would have ordered. Appropriately called 'hunter-gatherers' our early ancestors lived primarily off fruits, berries, roots and shoots and the occasional meat. But meat, their only acid food, formed only 20% or so of their diet.

Raw food

Ever since Hippocrates there have been those who advocate only the eating of raw foods. But what evidence is there that raw food is better for you? Firstly, our history suggests that we evolved to eat raw foods. After all, fire was only used by man in the last million years and even so it was primarily used to provide heat. Up until that time all food, including meat, was eaten raw.

Cooking also destroys nutrients. The greatest losses occur to vitamins B and C when food is boiled in water. These vitamins and also minerals leach out into water. The longer the food is boiled the more vitamins and minerals are lost. Pressure cooking, steaming or microwaving foods for as short a time as possible minimizes these losses. Microwaving vibrates water molecules within food which results in minimal water loss, and therefore minimal losses of water soluble vitamins and minerals. Fat soluble vitamins are destroyed by frying, since foods reach their highest temperature with this method of cooking. Also heated oils produce oxides which use up antioxidant vitamins A, C and E. The chart opposite summarizes the extensive losses of nutrients in foods when cooked.

Cooking doesn't only destroy vitamins and minerals. Many special substances exist within raw food. For example, nuts, seeds and alfalfa sprouts contain 'saponins' a kind of fat that has been shown to keep down blood cholesterol levels, thus reducing the risk for heart diease. Also, the beneficial effects of many forms of fibre are partially destroyed by cooking.

Proponents of eating raw foods also argue that

	Food Type	Per cent Loss of Vitamin			
		A	E	C	B Complex
Frying					
	Eggs	—	—	—	25
	Meat	—	0	20	20
Baking					
	Cereals	—	—	—	20
Boiling					
	Cereals	—	—	—	40
	Eggs	—	—	—	10
	Eggs (poached)	—	—	—	20
	Milk (pasteurized)	—	20	50	10
	Meat	0	20	30	40
	Vegetables	—	—	20	30
Grilling					
	Meat	0	20	20	20
(— denotes figures unavailable)					

Chart 3.6.2 — *Losses of nutrients from cooking food*

all food contains enzymes which may assist in digestion of the food, and that these enzymes are also destroyed by cooking. If this were the case cooked foods would require much more work to be digested and would draw on the body's reserves of energy and nutrients, making cooked food less nutritious. Although as yet unproved, the role of enzymes in food is likely to be of significance.

However, not everything in raw food is good for you. Cabbage, chinese leaves, watercress, kale, brussel sprouts and mustard contain glucosides which suppress thyroid function, fortunately only in those who are iodine deficient. Avidin in raw egg white binds biotin making it unavailable to the body. Phytic acid mainly in the bran of wholegrains renders minerals less absorbable and raw meats contain undesirable micro-organisms that can cause food poisoning. All these factors are significantly reduced by cooking.

Low mucus-forming diets

Although not widely recognized as a diet, work by nutritionist Robert Gray has come up with dietary strategies for cleaning the colon. He suggests that certain foods are mucus-forming or encourage the body to produce mucus. Mucus-like substances are by their nature sticky and may produce more compacted faecal matter, 'gunking up' the colon and slowing down gastro-intestinal transit time. While this idea has yet to be proven it is the experience of many people that those foods listed below as highly mucus-forming do produce excessive mucus and are best avoided by those with mucus related problems.[10]

Highly mucus-forming	Mildly mucus-forming	Non-mucus-forming
Milk and cream	Soya beans	Vegetables
Cheese	Pulses	Fruits
Butter	Nuts	Sprouting seeds
Yogurt	Seeds	
Meat	Grains	
Fish		
Eggs		

Chart 3.6.3 — *Mucus-forming foods*

Preparing healthy food

In previous chapters we've looked at what constitutes a healthy diet. This chapter helps you put these principles into practice. It does not, however, provide recipes since there already exist many excellent health food recipe books.

Keeping your fat intake down

It is well worth remembering the approximate fat content of different foods, then with a little forethought it is easy to keep a low fat intake. Meat provides a lot of fat, even lean meat or chicken. Fish (grilled or baked — not fried) or chicken without its skin are the best animal proteins in terms of their fat levels. Vegetarian proteins can also be high in fat, particularly hard cheeses, so choose reduced-fat cheddar (health food shop varieties do not contain additives), cottage and curd cheese. Eggs are high in fat, although valuable for their other nutrients. They are best eaten in moderation boiled, poached or baked (for exmaple, in quiches) in preferences to frying. Nuts are another example of a food high in fat and also nutrients, which although good for you should not be eaten in excess.

Alternatives to frying

Grilling foods is preferable to frying. When sautéing vegetables for a casserole or pie, use half the fat you are used to, you will find the job is done just as well and you won't have to use lots of flour to soak up the extra fat. Once the vegetables start to sizzle add in a couple of table-spoons of water and put the lid on. This mixture of light frying and steaming brings out the flavours in food.

Protecting essential fats

Polyunsaturates get damaged by heat, so always store your vegetable oils in the fridge and don't keep nuts anywhere hot. When cooking with fat use butter or olive oil. Safflower and sunflower oils can be used in salad dressings.

Low fat salad dressings

You will need to experiment with different salad dressings. A good place to start is a basic French dressing — two parts oil (safflower, sunflower or olive) to one part cider or wine vinegar, to this add any of the following — mustard, fresh or dried herbs, freshly ground black pepper, crushed garlic, a little honey. To make the dressing creamy and lower fat add cottage cheese, yogurt or a combination of mayonnaise, yogurt and milk. Another good dressing can be made using orange juice and oil in equal quantities with pepper and a little mustard.

Making the most of vegetables

The most important point to remember when buying vegetables is that a good vegetable is a fresh vegetable. No-one will find limp yellowing kale appetizing, but who could refuse fresh, green, crisp kale sautéed in lemon juice and a little soy sauce with garlic? Ideally, buy organically grown vegetables.

If these are unavailable outside leaves should be washed carefully to remove any chemicals. Discard as few outside leaves as possible as they contain many valuable nutrients. When cooking vegetables they should be cooked for as short a time as possible (so there is still 'bite' in them) and in as little water as possible (steam in a steamer or use half an inch of water). Don't forget that vegetables are an excellent food and should be eaten in plentiful quantities.

How to make delicious salads

If cooked vegetabes are good for you, raw ones are even better. A good salad can consist of many different vegetables, here are a few ideas to be eaten in any combination — carrot, raw beetroot, radish, bean sprouts, lettuce (crispy varieties are nicer), cucumber, radichio, tomato, alfalfa sprouts, pepper, apple, spinach, carrot tops, raw corn on the cob (cut off the cob) and peas lightly cooked. To your raw vegetable combination you can add walnuts, almonds, raisins or other nuts or seeds. With a delicious dressing a good salad should be the major part of your meal.

Beansprouts

Growing your own beansprouts provides you with the freshest vegetables possible, available all the year round. Health food shops sell purpose made beansprouters, alternatively use a large jar with a J-cloth or gauze over the top held with a rubber band. Put a handful of pulses in the bottom of the jar, cover with the cloth, half fill the jar with water and drain out, repeat this procedure twice a day until beans are sprouted. The following beans make good sprouts — chick peas, green lentils, mung beans, alfalfa seeds and whole wheat grains.

Preparing beans and lentils

Beans and lentils are an excellent low fat source of protein and carbohydrate and should be regularly included in your diet. Lentils are quick to cook (15-20 minutes for red, 30-35 minutes for brown or continental and 40-45 minutes for green) and taste good as part of soups or cas-

seroles. Other pulses take longer to cook unless they are soaked overnight and cooked in a pressure cooker. Chick peas, red kidney beans and black-eyed beans are among the most popular. However, there are many to try. They can be used with other vegetables in casseroles or made into a paté with lemon juice, olive oil and garlic, this way, eaten with bread the quality of protein is improved.

Preparing whole grains

To keep your complex carbohydrate levels high, rice and other whole grains should play a large part of your diet. Brown rice is faster to cook than it used to be (new varieties have been developed). It is easy to overcook brown rice — a good guide is one part rice to two parts water, simmered for 25 minutes, the rice should still be chewy. Other whole grains to try are millet, whole wheat, buckwheat or a combination.

Bread and its alternatives

Wholemeal bread is an excellent convenience food, to add variety try baking soda bread using corn meal in place of wheat flour, rice cakes, oatcakes or rye bread (beware most rye bread is 10% rye flour, 90% refined white flour, however 100% rye bread is available and delicious).

Eat less meat and more vegetarian protein

Remember that many people eat too much protein. If you cut down on meat, restrict your cheese intake and regularly eat pulses you should be getting enough. You do get some protein from vegetables and whole grains.

Flavouring foods without salt

When weaning yourself off salt it is important to flavour foods adequately. Use plenty of garlic — even in dishes that do not traditionally use it. There are many vegetable stock cubes and paste and vegetable bouillion powders available in health food shops, Vecon is a particularly good one — a bean is boring without the addition of Vecon or something similar. Tomato purée (without added salt) is good for increasing flavour.

Fresh or dried herbs should also be used in liberal amounts.

Making sweets without sugar

For the odd occasion that you feel the need for something sweet it is better that you sweeten with fresh or dried fruit. Date paste can be made by slowly stewing dried dates and then mashing to a paste, this can be used to sweeten all kinds of cakes, biscuits or puddings. Mashed, fresh banana is also a good sweetening agent. To make a delicious dried fruit bar, combine almonds, oats and apricots or dates in a food processor and process until thoroughly chopped. Then slowly add water or fruit juice until it forms a ball. Roll out and cut into shapes.

Alternative drinks

When you discover the world of herb teas and coffee substitutes, plain old tea and coffee appear boring. There must be hundreds of different herb teas and their combinations, all very different and preferred by different people — try them until you find one you like. Coffee substitutes are fewer in number, however very good. There are basically two types, dandelion coffee (roasted root or instant) or various different roasted grains in an instant form. Again try different brands until you find one you like. You can also drink diluted juice or water.

There is no practical work in this section. Just put these principles into effect with your own diet.

CHAPTER 3.8

The anti-nutrients

—OVERVIEW—

Nutrition isn't just a matter of eating the right things. It's also about not ingesting the wrong things. These include pollutants, food additives, chemicals and drugs, as well as harmful food factors and the effects of cooking. Many of these substances act specifically as 'anti-nutrients' causing their damaging effect by preventing the positive action of a nutrient. Lead for example, interferes with calcium and zinc utilization, hence causing its damaging effects to brain function. The side-effects of many drugs can also be attributed to their anti-nutrient activity.

Pollutants are present in air, drinking water and food. These include toxic metals such as lead, cadmium, mercury, arsenic, copper and aluminium. All of these are now present in quantities significantly larger than those for which the human body was designed. In addition to these, we are exposed to carcinogens from car exhaust, industrial processes, other people's cigarettes and pesticides and fungicides sprayed on our food. The average person has one gallon of pesticides sprayed on the food they eat, and breathes in one gram of heavy metals per year.

Food additives are chemicals that are added to food to alter taste, appearance and shelf life. Most of these are synthetic substances. They are tested for safety using short-term animal studies in isolation. Hence both their long-term effect on health, and their effect in combination is largely unknown. A number of permitted additives have been shown to cause hyperactivity and other adverse reactions in a small number of sensitive children.

The use of drugs inevitably impairs nutritional status. Even aspirins increase the need for vitamin C and may increase allergic potential. The use of cortisone and other hormone based drugs, including oestrogen, upsets the control systems and interferes with a number of nutrients. Tranquillizers, anti-depressants and hypnotic drugs are probably the worst problem, with 46.7 million prescriptions per year to a population of 58 million. It is estimated that one million women in Britain are addicted to some form of medication. A further three million are dependent on alcohol.

Finally, food itself contains natural anti-nutrients. Bran, for example, is rich in phytic acid which inhibits mineral absorption. Parsnips contain psoralen, a powerful carcinogen, and red kidney beans contain the anti-nutrient lectin which is fortunately destroyed by cooking. Cooking itself is probably the biggest anti-nutrient factor. With the exception of meat, fish, eggs and beans which need to be cooked to destroy harmful bacteria or food factors, cooking destroys valuable nutrients.

—TOXIC METALS—

The whole world, including us, is made out of elements. Some of these elements are essential, like zinc and calcium. Others are toxic and may interfere with nutrients. Among the most common toxic elements — lead, mercury, copper (although also an essential nutrient) and aluminium — lead toxicity is the most prevalent.

Lead

Researchers at the California Institute of Technology have been monitoring changes in lead concentrations throughout the world — in ocean beds, soil samples and even snow. Their work shows that lead concentration, even in unpolluted Greenland, has risen between 500 and 1,000 times since prehistoric ages. This rise has largely been the result of the use of lead in car exhaust. There is now little doubt that many people, especially children, are exposed to dangerous levels of lead.[11]

Three research studies have all shown conclusively that levels of lead as low as 13mcg/dl can affect behaviour and lower intelligence in children. Since the average EEC lead level is 13mcg/dl it is possible that lead is damaging the minds of one in two children in the EEC. Let's examine the evidence.

Herbert Needleman, associate professor of child psychiatry, looked at a group of 2,146 children in first and second grade schools in Birmingham, USA. He examined lead concentrations in shed baby teeth, to obtain more long term levels than shown by a simple blood test. He then asked the school teachers to rate the behaviour of children they had taught for at least two months. This was done using a questionnaire designed to measure the teacher's rating of childen for a number of characteristics, shown in Figure 3.8.1.[12]

His results showed a clear relationship between lead concentrations and bad school behaviour, as rated by the teachers without any knowledge of the children's lead levels. Perhaps the most interesting result was that none of the high lead

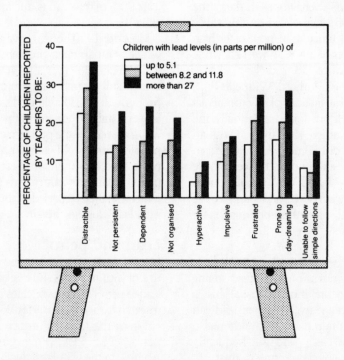

Figure 3.8.1 — *Needleman study*

children had an IQ above 125 points (100 is average), compared to 5% in the low lead group. .

Although Needleman's study shows that the behaviour and intelligence of normal children are clearly affected by lead, we cannot be sure of the severity of the problem in Britain. Nor can we determine safe blood levels for lead concentration, since his study used teeth.

Richard Lansdown, principal psychologist at the Hospital for Sick Children in London, and William Yule, psychologist at the University of London, decided to replicate the essentials of Needleman's study on London children, using blood lead levels instead of teeth. The children selected had an average blood lead level of 13.52mcg/dl (35mcg/dl is the 'safe' level recommended by the Lawther Report in 1980).[13]

Lansdown's results were even more striking than Needleman's. The difference in IQ score between high and low lead children was seven IQ points — even though none of the children had lead levels above 35mcg/dl, the 'safe' DHSS level. Their results showed that, around a blood lead level of 13mcg/dl, there is a clear adverse effect on children's behaviour. In fact, the 'threshold' level for safety based on this study would be 12mcg/dl. Once again, none of the high lead group children had IQs above 125, while in the low lead groups, 5% did.[14]

A further study of Gerhard Winneke PhD, director of the Medical Institute of Environmental Hygiene in Dusseldorf, found essentially the same results. He studied 458 children with an average blood level of 14.3mcg/dl, and found an IQ deficit of five to seven points between those with high and low lead levels. Winneke also looked at dentine (teeth) levels and found a close correlation to blood — a further confirmation for Needleman's results.[15]

Lead toxicity — who is at risk?

Although adults are not safe from lead poisoning it is children who are most at risk. This is especially so up to age twelve, when lead can create irreversible brain damage. Children also absorb lead more easily and are frequently exposed to higher concentrations in dust.

This means that a high proportion of children, particularly in cities are absorbing enough lead to affect their intellectual development. The most common symptoms in children are an inability to concentrate, disturbed sleep patterns, uncharacteristic aggressive outbursts, fussiness about food, sinus conditions and headaches. Children from birth to age eight are most at risk, with a peak around age two to three, although it is only the size of the problem that diminishes from age eight — the problem doesn't disappear. Adults are more likely to experience a chronic lack of physical and mental energy, together with headaches, depression and loss of memory.

Where does lead come from?

The immediate assumption is that lead comes directly from car exhausts. But this may not be the major source. A considerable quantity of lead from cars and lorries ends up on the food we eat. Whether it comes through milk, made by the cow that eats the grass by the motorway, or whether it comes directly from vegetables exposed to lead-polluted air, the result is too much lead in food. Most scientists agree that at least 90% of this lead is due to fall-out from car exhaust.

Most pre-1940 houses have some lead piping, which is a particular problem for those in soft water areas. However a greater problem is the solder still used in plumbing which, if not properly done is liable to dissolve. Paint is no longer a major source and the EEC regulations will soon reduce the problem even further. Only people stripping old paint for redecorating really run a risk. It is therefore best to remove such paint by using a steamer. This softens the paint, which can then be peeled off. Burning or scraping puts lead dust in the air.

Lead and petrol

Many countries have banned or restricted the use of lead in petrol. Russia banned the use of leaded petrol in its major cities in 1960, following research carried out in 1958. West Germany now enforces the lowest Europen levels of lead in petrol. The EPA (Environment Protection Agency) in the USA is gradually winning a leagal battle against the lead producing industry to further control the level of lead in fuel, which has been cut by half since 1976. This and other measures have caused a 30% drop in blood lead levels in the USA. Figure 3.8.2 shows the correlation between declining use of lead in petrol and average blood lead levels from 1976 to 1980.

Detoxifying lead

Once ingested lead must compete with other minerals for absorption. These minerals are called lead antagonists and form our first line of defence. Once the lead is absorbed, some natural body substances latch on to the lead and try to take it out of the body. These are called chelators (pronounced key-lay-tors). Vitamin C is a strong chelator of lead, while calcium helps to prevent its uptake.

Another substance known to lower lead is zinc which acts as an antagonist to lead by preventing its absorption in the gut. One study by Carl Pfeiffer Ph.D.[16] administered 2,000mg of vitamin C and 60mg of zinc (as zinc gluconate) to 22 workers at a lead battery plant, all of whom had elevated lead levels. After 24 weeks there was a striking decrease in lead levels despite no change in exposure. A supplement containing zinc, calcium and vitamin C, called *Detox*, is available from Health + Plus Ltd. (Phone: 0844 52098) as a means for promoting the elimination of lead and protecting from its absorption.

Mercury

Mercury is one of the most toxic elements known to man. Fortunately mercury poisoning is extremely rare and is usually the result of occupational exposure. The early warnings signs of toxicity include forgetfulness, fatigue and headaches. These are important to detect since the clinical symptoms, tingling, headaches, visual, hearing and speech defects, paralysis and convulsions, are irreversible. However many of us are inadvertently exposed to small amount of mercury from amalgam fillings and from fish.

Mercury in fillings

Mercury has been used in dental fillings for over

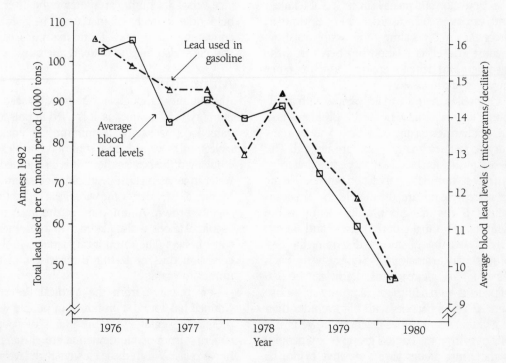

Figure 3.8.2 — *Decreased use of lead in petrol* vs *blood lead*

150 years because 'when mercury is combined with the metals used in dental amalgam, its toxic properties are made harmless' says the American Dental Association.[17] However, with the advent of highly sensitive modern detection equipment, there is now evidence to show that highly toxic mercury can migrate from teeth fillings to other parts of the body, causing a whole range of health problems in a small number of susceptible individuals.

To fill a cavity a dentist produces a mixture of silver, copper, zinc, tin and mercury. The cavity is then lined with a resin liner to supposedly seal the cavity and then the amalgam is added. This method would be quite acceptable if the mercury stayed in place within the filling. Between 1970 and 1982 five different researchers have all found astonishing losses of mercury ranging from 53% to 84%.[18]

Once out of the tooth, the potential for damage is extensive. It acts as a 'brain poison' causing both motor disorders, similar to multiple sclerosis, in addition to emotional disturbances like depression and mental illness. It is also linked with cardiovascular disorders and deformity in pregnancy. Yet it is almost impossible to show a cause and effect relationship between these disorders and dental mercury. Too many other variables are involved.

Obviously there are many people with amalgam fillings who have no health problems and are not harmed in any noticeable way by mercury. So just how many people are affected? The dental profession has always accepted that there is a tiny section of the population who are allergic to mercury and are unsuitable for amalgam fillings. But is this group quite so tiny as the dentists try to make out? Djerassi and Berova carried out a unique study to determine the level of sensitivity to amalgam.[18] Subjects were patch tested for allergic reactions to amalgam. 16.1% of patients with fillings gave a positive response and 22.5% of patients with fillings older than five years had a positive reaction. However not one person in the control group (sixty people) without any fillings gave a positive response. These findings suggest that for many people mercury is escaping from their fillings and they are unable to accommodate this added toxic burden.

Mercury in fish

The Minamata Bay disaster in Japan, in which 700 people were mercury poisoned, 46 of which died, highlighted the danger of industrial compounds contaminating fish. Mercury-based compounds, used in many pesticides, fungicides, paints, cosmetics and batteries, still find their way into rivers and oceans. In the Minamata Bay disaster only ten to twenty parts per million (ppm) of mercury were found in the contaminated bay water, as a result of industrial waste. This reduced to 0.5ppm when the source of pollution was stopped. Levels of mercury greater than 20ppm have already been found in fish caught off the coast of Britain. Deep sea fish and frozen fish, often caught in distant waters, are less likely to be so contaminated.

Detoxifying mercury

Mercury is strongly antagonistic to selenium and vice versa. Selenium can therefore be given to help rid the body of mercury. The sulphur containing amino acids, found in onions, garlic and eggs, also help to detoxify mercury.

Aluminium

Aluminium, although not as toxic as lead or mercury, is all around us. It is used in pots and pans, food packaging, aluminium foil, antacid tablets and is even added to some foods to bleach, emulsify or help raise them. It is also added to water in areas high in peat, as it helps remove humic acid, rendering the water clear rather than slightly brown. Aluminium, in the form of a 'sacrificial anode' is also placed in many domestic water boilers. The aluminium sacrifices itself to corrosion thus protecting the surfaces of the immersion tank.

New research from the Medical Research Council has found aluminium in people with premature senility.[19] In the brains of people suffering from senile dementia are clusters of nerve cells. Within these clusters high levels of aluminium are often found. First identified by Dr Pfeiffer of the Brain Bio Center more than fifteen years ago, the true dangers of aluminium are at last being taken seriously. Mental ability declines in women and men from the age of fifty and the incidence of senile dementia has reached epidemic proportions, affecting more than 250,000 people.

Detoxifying aluminium
It is relatively easy to avoid or at least minimize exposure to aluminium from food packaging and cooking utensils. Calcium and magnesium are also thought to help keep aluminium levels to a minimum.

Additives and preservatives
By far the most important source of anti-nutrients and undesirable chemicals is the food we eat. Whether high in additives or preservatives or sprayed with pesticides, the fact that these chemicals are eaten means that we must be extra careful to ensure that they are safe. And many of them are not, as Sophie's story tells.

Sophie, age two, was one of twenty children chosen to take part in a test for sensitivity to food colourings. For six months she was strictly kept away from any foods with colourings or salicy-lates (found in aspirin, cherries and plums). Then, without her or her mother knowing what was being added, Dr Weiss added on some days dummy substances, and other days small amounts of food colourings most commonly added to our foods. Whenever the food colour-ings were added Sophie changed . . . like Jekyll and Hyde. She started throwing and breaking things, whining and running away and was clearly unwell. On these occasions her mother guessed she'd been given colourings. In fact, over seventy-seven days she was given colourings six times. Her mother guessed right five times. When the daily dose was increased no less than seventeen out of twenty children showed the same changes in behaviour.[20]

These results alerted mothers and doctors to the problems of food additives, but no action was taken to restrict the colouring agents or even publicize the facts. Now, five years later, researchers from the Institute for Child Health and the Hospital for Sick Children in London

have confirmed these results. They studied seventy-six 'overactive' children. Sixty-two improved on a diet free from additives. Forty-eight different foods were found to cause a reaction and artificial colourings and preserva-tives were found to be the commonest provoking substances.

No action is being taken by the government or the food industry to ban the use of these colourings, although the new labelling laws introducing 'E' numbers, with a little guidance, will make the art of chemical self-defence much easier. In line with EEC regulations, all food additives are now allocated an E number. For the manufacturers, this means they won't have to put long lists of chemical sounding ingredients on their products . . . just long lists of E numbers, if they choose to use them.

But how do we break the E numbers code? First of all, different types of additives form different E number series, for example colouring agents are numbered between E100 and E180. Here are the rest:

Preservatives	E200 to E290
Anti-oxidants	E300 to E330
Emulsifiers	E322 to E495
Sweeteners	E420 to E421
Solvents	E422
Mineral hydrocarbons	E905 to E907

But do we really need any of these? Let's concern ourselves with the first four categories. Colours are added to make our food look good. Of course, if you don't mind eating peas that don't glow in the dark and can accept that haddock isn't naturally bright yellow, then it is better to avoid all food colours. E102, Tartrazine, is a widely-used orange/yellow colouring which has been shown to cause hyperactivity. See *The New E for Additives* by Maurice Hanssen (Thorsons, 1987) for further details.

Preservatives prevent the growth of micro-organisms like mould. Often the effects of mould are far worse than the effects of preservatives. However, if you can buy food fresh that's the best. It's a matter of choice. Sausages, for example contain nitrates (E250-E252) to prevent some very dangerous micro-organisms. But the more nitrates you eat the more you risk forming nitro-samines, which are potent cancer producing chemicals. There are no preservatives that are actually good for you.

Anti-oxidants stop food becoming rancid. This is most important for fats and oils. Nature equips foods with anti-oxidants. Seeds, high in oils, are also high in vitamin E. Vitamin E is a good anti-oxidant. Its E numbers are E306, E307, E308 and E309. Another natural anti-oxidant is vitamin C. Its E numbers are E300, E301, E302, E303 and E304. Other anti-oxidants like BHA (E320) and BHT (E321) are of dubious safety.

Emulsifiers help to bind and emulsify sauces. It's the lecithin in egg that makes mayonnaise what it is. Lecithin is E322. Other emulsifiers like the polyphosphates, E450, are there so that more water can be added to meats, increasing the company's profits.

Pesticides

In 1985 3,000 incidents of illness resulting from pesticide poisoning were recorded — including one death. A survey by the Ministry of Agri-culture, Foods and Fisheries found that between 97% and 99% of all fresh fruit, cereals and vegetables are sprayed with pesticides. That means that most meat and milk is contaminated from pesticides used on the animal's food. Although few proper surveys have been carried out to find the size of the problem the Association of Public Analysts are gravely concerned. In 1983 they randomly tested 305 fruits. Thirty-one of these samples contained levels of pesticides above the levels deemed safe, and a further seventy-two samples showed lower pesticide levels. Some fruits, particularly strawberries, raspberries, grapes and tomatoes had measurable levels of at least six different pesticides!

Even more alarming was the fact that some of the pesticides found are not 'cleared for use' in Britain, while others, although permitted, are banned in many other countries because of their known damage to health, promoting cancer and causing birth defects. One of these, DDT, has been banned. However a further survey by the Public Analysts found that, out of 293 samples of different fruits and vegetables 10% contained DDT! It is clear that DDT is still in widespread, if illicit use.

One billion gallons of pesticides are sprayed on to our foods each year, many of which are of dubious necessity. Often there are far safer alternatives. for example, organophosphorus compounds are sprayed on to stored grains to stop insect damage. These products are patent-able, hence profitable. They also don't do the job very well, because in time, the insects develop tolerance and some new chemical must be intro-duced. But merely storing the grain in a carbon dioxide rich environment deprives the insects of oxygen and protects the crop at a margin of the cost. The more pesticides are used, the more resistant the insects become so the more pesti-cides have to be used. It's a vicious circle.

Companies like ICI sell billions of gallons of pesticides every year. Many of these sales are to third world countries who have few restrictions on their use. Since there are no controls governing the importation of foods sprayed with 'illegal' pesticides, these in turn end up on our plates. But not all the blame can be put on the chemical industry. Farmers are, in many instances, blissfully unaware of how to use pesticides correctly and what their dangers are. Many of the 'casualties' reported from pesticide exposure include farm workers who didn't wear protective clothing, and people living downwind from a farm engaged in spraying.

So what can you do? Firstly, more and more shops are stocking organically grown pesticide free food. These can sometimes be found in greengrocers, health food shops and super-markets. Try to get food that conforms to the standards set by the Soil Association and the British Organic Farmers. All foods that are grown organically are pesticide free.

If you live in the country try smallholdings selling home-grown vegetables. Ask them what they use. Often this local produce is pesticide free. Alternatively, grow your own. If you live in the town you can let your greengrocer know that you'd rather buy pesticide free food. Most markets have organic and pesticide free food, so the greengrocers can get it if they want to. Sometimes it's a little more expensive, but so much tastier. Failing that, the best you can do is to wash fruit and vegetables. Putting vinegar in the water helps to remove pesticides as well as toxic metals like lead. Boiling foods also helps to break down the chemicals.

Nitrates

Another type of anti-nutrients of grave concern is nitrates and nitrites. Due to the overuse of nitrates in fertilizers for the past forty years levels of nitrates in food, water and soil have now reached dangerous levels. The danger is caused by the fact that nitrates can turn into nitrites, and nitrites can combine with amines to produce nitrosamines, one of the strongest cancer producing chemicals known to man.

Since nitrates used in farming have now seeped into the water table there is no way of avoiding them completely. The main source of nitrate intake is vegetables (more than 70% of total intake) followed by water (21%) followed by meat.

Drugs — do you really need them?

As a nation, our consumption of medical drugs is the highest in the world. The British pharmaceutical industry turn over a staggering £2,000 million a year. But do we really need to take this many? In many instances the answer is no. For example, the use of aspirin for mild pain and headaches can never do us any long term good. The human body has no need for its active ingredient 'salicylic acid'. Continual use of aspirin is known to increase risk of stomach ulceration and kidney disease, as well as blocking vitamin C uptake and lowering folic acid levels. In 1980 the 6th World Nutrition Congress reported that even a single aspirin can make your intestines bleed for a week![21]

Some people take caffeine-based pain killers, since coffee drinkers deprived of coffee will suffer headaches as a sign of withdrawal. Out of the frying pan into the fire! Vitamin B_3 in the niacin (or nicotinic acid) form often relieves headaches and even migraines by causing a dilation of blood vessels. Doses of between 100 and 400mg are recommended. But watch out, because you'll blush and go a little hot and itchy for about 20 minutes as your blood vessels dilate. This effect is good for you, but not everybody likes it.

Another common and extremely dangerous drug is cortisone. Cortisone is a synthetic form of the hormone produced by the adrenal gland to combat stress. This substance has almost magical qualities in that it can reduce pain, stop inflammatory reactions, prevent transplanted organs being rejected, and is now used to treat over 100 different ailments including cancer, arthritis, kidney disease, hay fever and allergies. In America 29 million prescriptions for it are written each year! 'The sad truth is that cortisone doesn't cure anything: it merely suppresses the symptoms of the disease', say Dr Zumoff, formerly with the Steroid Research Laboratory at New York's Montefiore Hospital.[22] One of the major problems with this drug is that the body stops producing its own cortisone. Suddenly stopping cortisone can therefore result in collapse with a rapid fall of blood-pressure and a real danger of death. It can take over two years for the adrenal glands to start producing this hormone again after long term use of cortisone. Other side effects include a rounded face, increase in fat deposits, greater risk of infection, poor wound healing and a greater risk of congestive heart failure and kidney disease.

One of the most dangerous aspects of many drugs is the fact that no two people will necessarily react in the same way. Professor Smoth at St Mary's Hospital in London believes that one in every ten people has a faulty metabolism which can result in abnormal drug reactions.

> Often a poor metabolizer needs less than a quarter of the normal dose. I think we are going to find many more genetic differences and many more drugs that are affected. Until now adverse reactions were blamed on the drug. I think from now on we will be looking far more at the individual and how he or she handles the drug.

The chart below shows some of the known effects drugs have on compromising good nutrition. Wherever possible drugs are best avoided.

HOW DRUGS DEPLETE VITAMINS AND MINERALS	
B$_1$ thiamine	Antibiotics, oral contraceptives
B$_2$ riboflavine	Antibiotics
B$_6$ pyridoxine	Steroid hormones, cortisone
B$_{12}$ cyanocobalamine	Antibiotics, anti-tuberculosis
Biotin	Antibiotics, sulphur drugs
Folic acid	Oral contraceptives, diuretics
Inositol	Antibiotics
C	Aspirin, corticosteroids, oral contraceptives
D	Anticonvulsants
E	Oral contraceptives
K	Antiobiotics, anticoagulants, aspirin
Zinc	Oral contraceptives
Copper	Oral contraceptives
Potassium	Diuretics

Chart 3.8.1 — *Drug-nutrient interactions*

Coffee

Caffeine belongs to a large and diverse group of naturally occurring chemicals known as alkaloids. Alkaloids have been used for thousands of years for social, medical and religious reasons and their effects can vary from mild stimulation and hallucinatory effects to inhibition and even death. Thus it is not surprising to find out that many drugs, including morphine and quinine, are alkaloids. The effects of most alkaloids is dose related and small quantities are usually tolerated without problems.

Two strong cups of coffee can, in some cases, have an observable toxic effect. These symptoms are indistinguishable from anxiety and are frequently misdiagnosed as problems of psychological origin. They include restlessness, nervousness, flushed face, insomnia and even cardiovascular complications such as rapid pulse and palpitations.

Coffee is also addictive. Like any stimulant it is easy to become relatively dependent on coffee's stimulating effect. As the endocrine system becomes stressed by regular use of stimulants as time goes on more or stronger coffee is needed for the same effect. This leads, literally, to addiction, until the coffee drinker cannot go without coffee without experiencing withdrawal effects including lack of energy and headaches.

Unfortunately this is not the limit to coffee's detrimental effects. Coffee also contains a number of suspected and proven carcinogens. Caffeine has been shown to increase the production of cancer tumours in animals and there is now evidence to suggest that heavy coffee drinking is associated with cancer. Methylxanthines found in coffee breaks down to produce free radicals which are linked with both cancer and premature ageing. In addition coffee drains the body of vital nutrients. Iron, zinc, calcium and magnesium have all be shown to have reduced rates of absorption or increased rates of excretion when food containing these minerals is taken with coffee. So if you are going to drink coffee it is best to take it away from meal times.

Although an improvement, decaffeinated coffee is not the answer. It still contains some stimulants and other nasties linked with cancer. The best option is to leave the coffee bean well alone and adopt alternatives such as Barleycup, dandelion coffee or herb teas like the Celestial Seasonings range.

Alcohol

Alcohol is a potent drug that anaesthetizes the brain. In the cortex area of the brain, it acts as a relaxant and too much distorts learning ability, memory, control, judgement and behaviour. But it doesn't just affect the brain. All cells are exposed to alcohol, especially the liver and kidneys. The blood vessels in the kidneys dilate, causing frequent urination, and the cells in the liver become damaged and scarred. There is no doubt that long term use of alcohol causes inflammation and scarring (cirrhosis) of the liver and also increases the chances of kidney disease.

How much is too much?

One study investigated decreased alcohol consumption as the possible cause for slight decreases in blood-pressure for patients staying in hospital. To test their theories they equipped a group of in-patients with a can of beer each day and sure enough their blood-pressure didn't decline. However, not all agree that total abstinence is the best thing for the heart and arteries. One astonishing finding is that moderate alcohol consumption actually increases high-density lipoprotein, the carrier that takes cholesterol out of the arteries. Moderate means one ounce a day, that is two beers or two glasses of wine.[23] However those with a history of moderately high blood-pressure can do well to avoid alcohol at any time as it is well established that alcohol is a major contributor to hypertension. Alcohol consumption also increases the risk of many other illnesses including cancer and mental illness.

Alcohol — the anti-nutrient

Many of alcohol's harmful effects can be attributed to its action as an anti-nutrient. Drinkers tend to have depleted levels of many vitamins and minerals, especially vitamin A, all the Bs, C, magnesium, zinc and essential fatty acids. Most of all alcohol consumption badly affects the availability of zinc. Research at Oregon State University has revealed that consumption of alcohol, while on a zinc-sufficient diet, produces zinc deficiency, equivalent to that of a zinc-deficient diet without any alcohol. So alcohol is a powerful anti-zinc factor. It also promotes the absorption of lead. According to Alan Knowles, Director of the Westminster Advisory Centre on Alcoholism, 'Almost all our clients have high levels of lead in the hair. I believe the effects of lead poisoning and alcohol poisoning are all intertwined.'[24] It's a vicious circle because the more one is exposed to lead the more this excites the nervous system, making alcohol, a relaxant, particularly appealing. But while the alcohol does help in the short term it increases the absorption of lead. Both lead and alcohol are known to increase aggressive behaviour, and both are frequently found to be high in criminals and hooligans.[25]

Nutritional help for alcoholics

According to Dr Carl Pfeiffer,[26] the problem drinker can be fitted into four major types. These are: the compulsive, depressed hard-core drinker, who tends to produce too much histamine; the weekend belligerent binge drinker, who may be low in histamine and high in copper, the 'allergic' drinker with an allergy to hops, yeast, malt or grains; and the hypoglycaemic drinker who substitutes alcohol for sugar.

The use of megavitamins both for reducing cravings and speeding up the physical and mental recovery of alcoholics is well proven. Particularly important are large doses of vitamin C (5 to 10 grams daily) and vitamin B_3 (100-500mg). But these aren't all. The high-histamine drinker needs more calcium and B_6 which help to lower excess histamine. 90% of alcoholics fall into this group. These people are very prone to depression and use alcohol, often unconsciously, as a means for slow suicide. The amino acid methionine also lowers excess histamine.

But the greatest danger that alcohol poses is to the unborn child. This topic is discussed in chapter 5.3.

Nutrition and smoking

The dangerous effects of smoking on the health of the smoker may not occur for many years. Many people say that they will stop smoking when they reach a certain age, but every single cigarette causes substantial damage. Most of all smoking increases the risk of lung cancer, lung diseases and heart disease. Over 90% of all deaths from lung cancer are attributed to smoking and the highest incidence of lung cancer is in men aged sixty-five to seventy-four who smoked heavily during World War 2. In this age group over 500 pople in every 100,000 die from lung cancer. While stopping smoking does reduce the risk of developing cancer (by 80% after fifteen years abstinence) the primary factor in deciding your risk is the total length of one's smoking life.

Cigarettes contain numerous toxins, including nicotine, benzopyrene and the high intake of carbon monoxide as a function of burning tobacco. Nicotine is the primary addictive component but benzopyrene and carbon monoxide are most damaging to body cells, damaging the cell's DNA, causing it to mutate into a cancer cell. Nutrition can help to reduce the damaging effects of cigarettes and effect a speedier recovery by mopping up the free radicals caused by smoking, and by boosting the immune system to contain and destroy existing cancer cells. We all produce a potential cancer cell every day but, with a strong immune system, it doesn't stand a chance. The minerals selenium, zinc, copper and manganese are needed in disarming free radicals and so are vitamins E and C. This helps to restore immune function depleted by smoking.

PART FOUR

HEALTH AND NUTRITION

CHAPTER 4.1

Nutrition for a healthy heart

—OVERVIEW—

Coronary heart disease is the most common cause of death in western society, killing more than one in every three people. A heart attack occurs when the blood supply to the heart muscle is stopped and the heart is starved of oxygen. When the same process occurs in the brain this is called a stroke. So both a heart attack and a stroke are diseases of the arteries.

There are three stages of arterial damage that precede both a heart attack and a stroke. In the first stage, cells in the middle layer of the arterial wall mutate and proliferate. This is thought to be caused by circulating free radicals. Free radicals are dangerous chemicals caused by pollutants, particularly those in tobacco and polyunsaturated fats that have gone rancid. This type of cell proliferation is very similar to the development of cancer.

The mass of mutated cells then attracts cholesterol and other matter from the blood and a plaque or atheroma develops. This has the effect of narrowing the artery. Cholesterol is transported through the blood by two different types of carrier, known as low density lipoproteins (LDLs) and high density lipoproteins (HDLs). Cholesterol carried by LDLs is deposited in the artery wall but HDL cholesterol is transported to the liver for breakdown. Thus HDL cholesterol is beneficial and reduces the risk of heart disease.

In the final stage a clot forms, either due to a piece of plaque breaking away or because the blood has become excessively sticky, which blocks the already narrowed artery resulting in a stroke or heart attack.

Numerous nutritional or non-nutritional factors have been linked with an increased risk of heart disease. The non-nutritional factors include smoking, a lack of exercise, stress, and a competitive, time pressured personality, known as type A. Nutritional factors include an excess of dietary fats, refined sugar and salt and a deficiency of vitamins and minerals, especially vitamin E, selenium and magnesium.

British people have the second highest risk of heart disease in the world.[27] Literally thousands of women and men die prematurely every year usually between the ages of forty-five and sixty-five. However heart disease and strokes are also the second major cause of death in people between the ages of thirty-five and forty-five.

The incidence of heart disease has increased dramatically since the beginning of this century which points to changes in diet or lifestyle as being the most likely cause. Before exploring the cause of cardiovascular disease let us examine the nature of the problem.

Understanding cardiovascular disease

The major cause for death from arterial disease results from the blockage of arteries, resulting in the lack of blood, and hence oxygen, to cells in the body. Such blockages are in part the result of the build up of arterial plaque, known as atheromas, a disease called atherosclerosis (sclerosis means scarring). If a blockage occurs in the arteries supplying the heart with oxygen this can cause a heart attack or myocardial infarction. A slight blockage may result in angina, normally resulting in chest pain on exertion, as the heart is deprived of sufficient oxygen. If the blockage occurs in blood vessels in the head this causes one type of stroke, resulting in death or partial paralysis due to oxygen deprivation for some part of the brain. (A stroke can also be caused by haemorrhage of the fragile arteries in the brain.)

The existence of a blockage is usually the result both of atherosclerosis and the existence of clots in the blood, called thrombosis. A presence of large clots in the legs is called thrombophlebitis, and in the lungs is called a pulmonary embolism. In addition, arteries often lose their elasticity and become harder, which is called arteriosclerosis.

Next to these is the life expectancy that life insurance companies predict when your blood-pressure is low.

High blood-pressure itself does not diagnose atherosclerosis since this can be caused by a change in either blood viscosity or changes in the muscle tension surrounding arteries. The electrolyte minerals, sodium, potassium, calcium and magnesium all influence blood-pressure. Sodium raises blood-pressure while potassium, calcium and magnesium lower it. The relatively recent discovery that a muscular spasm in the coronary artery can cause a heart attack has made many cardiologists question how commonly heart attacks may be caused by this, rather than atherosclerosis.

The blood fats that predict heart disease

As well as monitoring your blood-pressure the presence of cholesterol, triglycerides and certain lipoproteins in the blood are good predictors of

AGE		> 35		35-55		55+	
		Men	Women	Men	Women	Men	Women
Healthy	120/80	76.5	?	77	82	78.5	82.5
Acceptable	130/90	72.5	?	74	79.5	77.5	82
Borderline	140/95	67.5	?	71	77	74.5	79.5
Hypertension	150/100	60	?	65.5	73.5	72.5	78.5

Chart 4.1.1 — *Blood-pressure and life expectancy*

Hypertension

All these problems affect the pressure in the arteries. When one's blood-pressure becomes raised this is called hypertension. Although hypertension can be caused by reasons other than atherosclerosis, monitoring blood-pressure is of crucial importance in preventing cardiovascular disease. The acceptable level for blood pressure is a hotly disputed issue. Some doctors allow a systolic (top) blood pressure of 100 plus your age, while others point out that in some cultures blood-pressure doesn't rise significantly with age. The above guidelines provide an indication of acceptable blood-pressure scores.

cardiovascular disease. When fats have been digested and absorbed they are put into the form of triglycerides. An excessive consumption of fat, or sugar which can be turned into fat, will raise triglyceride levels. Cholesterol, although no longer thought to be such an important factor in the diet, can become raised in the blood and is thought to speed up the process of atherosclerosis.

Cholesterol, being a constituent of bile, is released in the digestive system to help with digestion, and most is then reabsorbed and passes back to the liver, the rest being excreted in the faeces. Cholesterol in the walls of the arteries is carried in the blood to the liver by means of a substance called high density lipoprotein (HDL). Low HDL levels and high total cholesterol levels are strongly associated with atherosclerosis. But what actually causes cardiovascular disease?

The cholesterol myth

In 1913 a Russian scientist, Dr Anitschkov, thought he had found the answer to heart disease when he found that feeding cholesterol to rabbits induced heart disease.[28] However, there are some problems in comparing what happens in a vegetarian animal with what happens in man. Since the fatty deposits in the arteries of people with heart disease have been found to be high in cholesterol, it was soon thought that these deposits were the result of an excess of cholesterol in the blood, possibly caused by an excess of cholesterol in the diet.

Such a simple theory has its attractions and many doctors advocate a low cholesterol diet as the answer to heart disease. But controversy reigns in this area; see Pincbey's book *The Cholesterol Controversy,* (Sherbourne Press, 1973).

Dr Alfin-Slater from the University of California decided to test the cholesterol theory: 'We, like everyone else, had been convinced that when you eat cholesterol, you get cholesterol. When we stopped to think, none of the studies in the past had tested what happens to cholesterol levels when eggs — high in cholesterol — were added to a normal diet.'[29]

They selected fifty healthy people with normal blood cholesterol levels. Half of them were given two eggs per day (in addition to the other cholesterol rich foods they were already eating as part of their normal diet) for eight weeks. The other half were given one extra egg per day for four weeks, then two extra eggs per day for the next four weeks. Result — no change in blood cholesterol. Later, Dr Alfin-Slater commented: 'Our findings surprise us as much as ever . . .'

Three other studies (Professor Ismail, 1976;[30] Dr Hirshowitz, 1976;[30] Dr Herbert, 1977[31]) found no rise in blood cholesterol levels. In fact, as long ago as 1974 a British advisory panel set up by the government to look at 'Medical aspects of food policy on diet related to cardiovascular

disease' issued this statement: 'Most of the dietary cholesterol in western communities is derived from eggs, but we have found no evidence which relates the number of eggs consumed to the risk of heart disease.'[32]

During the height of cholesterol phobia, Dr Jolliffe, renowned for his weight-reducing diets, started an anti-coronary club and placed 814 men, aged forty to fifty-nine and all free from heart disease, on a low cholesterol, high polyunsaturate diet. For a control group, he had 463 men of similar age and health status, who continued with a normal (and thus relatively high cholesterol) diet. Five years later, eight men on the low cholesterol diet had died from heart attacks, compared with none from those in the control group![33] Ironically, Dr Jollife himself died from 'vascular complications of diabetes' at the age of fifty-nine, so he never lived to see the results.

Are fats to blame?

As scientists became disillusioned with the cholesterol diets the attention turned to saturated fat. After all, eating too much fat does lead to obesity and the incidence of heart disease in obese people is twice as high. Too much saturated fat does raise blood levels of triglycerides and also blood cholesterol, both of which are good indicators of a high risk. Also, the fatty streaks and deposits that occur in arteries are high in cholesterol with some triglycerides. Fats and cholesterol are also generally present in the same food. Although a high saturated fat diet does appear to be a risk factor for cardiovascular disease research has not been convincing in categorically blaming fat consumption for arterial disease.

With the saturated fat and cholesterol theories being widely accepted many people switched to eating polyunsaturated oils. Although an overall reduced intake of fat, and a relative increase in polyunsaturated oils is consistent with health, many people simply substituted polyunsaturated for saturated fat. Since polyunsaturates, especially when heated or not extracted by cold-press methods are particularly prone to oxidation it is not surprising that some studies showed an increase in cancer and premature ageing among those eating large quantities of polyunsaturates.

How fish oil protects against heart disease

At least one kind of polyunsaturated oil has been shown to have a protective effect on heart disease. Eicosapentaenoic acid (or EPA for short), found in oily fish, has been shown to lower triglycerides and, to a lesser extent, cholesterol, raise HDLs and thin the blood. It is these properties which are thought to have protected the Eskimos, whose diet is rich in cholesterol and saturated fat, from cardiovascular disease.

New theories of heart disease

Although much has been learnt about cardio-vascular disease no single explanation, dietary or otherwise fits all the facts. The presence of cholesterol and fats within the arterial plaque is thought to have more to do with improper hand-ling of these substances rather than just excess. Within arterial plaque is also found cancer-like cells and there is some considerable evidence that damage to the arterial wall, probably by free oxidizing radicals as in cigarette smoke or heated fats, may cause a proliferation of abnormal cells which possibly accumulate cholesterol. Once the atheroma starts to develop a second change occurs in the artery with the formation of a fibrous plaque. This is rich in calcium and one postulated theory is that these processes are a response to injury of the arterial wall — a puncture repair mechanism, if you like.

There are many risk factors for heart disease

Whatever the actual mechanism that causes the build up of atheromas there is no doubt that there are many dietary and lifestyle factors that increase your risk for heart disease.

The risk factors for cardiovascular disease (*in order of likely importance*)

Family history of cardiovascular disease
High blood lipids
High blood pressure
Smoking
Overweight
Lack of exercise
Chronic stress
Too much fat, sugar and salt
Deficiency in vitamins and minerals

Chart 4.1.2 — *Risk factors in heart disease*

If cardiovascular disease or diabetes runs in the family then it is likely other family members will be prone to high fat levels in the blood. However the presence of such a genetic weakness doesn't mean cardiovascular problems will develop as long as other risk factors are not present.

Smokers have a 70% higher risk for cardio-vascular disease. Smoking increases atherosclero-sis, and encourages blood clotting. Carbon monoxide, among other damaging substances in cigarettes, may cause damage to the artery walls, triggering off the processes that lead to artery disease. On stopping smoking there is an immediate reduction in risk, probably because the blood clotting effects of smoking may, in many cases be the 'final straw'. Aften ten years of no smoking a smoker has much the same risk as a non-smoker. Pipe or cigar smokers don't have anything like the risk of cigarette smokers.

While being 20% over your ideal weight predisposes you to cardiovascular problems slight excessive weight does not. (See Ideal Weight chart in Chapter 4.7) The incidence of angina is greatly increased in overweight people. Tied in with obesity is exercise. Regular exercise improves the health of the whole cardiovascular system and has been shown to lower cholesterol. Inactive people often put on weight later in life as their metabolism slows down, making exerise of some sort a critical factor. Also, people who exercise have been shown to have a relatively reduced appetite for food.

The role of stress in heart disease is often

overstated. The claim is often made that 'type A' people, the striving, competitive, impatient, workaholic and slightly hostile person over-committed to their vocation is more at risk. However, as a chairman of a multinational company once said 'I don't get ulcers. I give them'. Often people who are put under constant pressure and have difficulty saying 'no' become equally stressed and anxious. Stress in any form does deplete the body of vital vitamins and minerals, particularly zinc, magnesium, vitamin C and B vitamins, as well as suppressing the immune system. These, and other stress 'characteristics' including smoking and drinking, may explain in part why stress is connected with cardiovascular disease.

Vitamins that protect against heart disease

The two most important nutrients for a healthy heart are vitamins E and C. According to researchers Drs Wilfrid and Evan Shute vitamin E protects against heart disease in six ways.[34] It prevents blood clots forming in the arteries and helps dissolve existing clots. It increases the blood's supply of oxygen by helping red blood cells to transport oxygen. Therefore it enables the heart to pump more effectively on less oxygen. It prevents excessive scarring of the heart after a heart attack, and it is a dilator of the capillaries, improving cells' permeability for nutrients.

The beneficial effects of vitamin E have been shown in two large surveys to be most effective when doses in excess of 400iu are taken each day. In one study of 2,508 people between the ages of fifty and ninety-eight, who had taken 400iu or more each day for ten years, there were only four incidents of heart disease as compared with the expected 836 that occur in the general population.[35]

However, there are some precautions. Some people with high blood pressure or rheumatic heart disease, if given a large initial dose of vitamin E, can experience raised blood pressure before it begins to reduce. Therefore it is a wise precaution to start supplementing vitamin E at a daily intake of 100iu and increase this gradually until the therapeutic dose of around 400 to 1,000iu is reached.

Vitamin C is also critical in the prevention of heart disease. Collagen, the 'intercellular glue' that keeps arteries supple, depends upon vitamin C. A lack of vitamin C can also make arteries more permeable and prone to damage. Being an anti-oxidant vitamin C protects against free radical damage. Many studies have shown low levels of vitamin C in heart attack patients. This may be connected with stress or indeed smoking, both of which greatly deplete this essential vitamin. But more controversial is vitamin C's role in lowering high cholesterol levels. Research started by Dr Ginter in Czechoslovakia has shown that supplementing 1,000mg of vitamin C lowers a high blood cholesterol level by anything from 5% to 20%. There is some suggestion that vitamin C actually helps to dissolve arterial plaques.[36] Another vitamin that has been shown to lower blood cholesterol levels is vitamin B_3.

Minerals that protect against heart disease

Working together with vitamin C and E is the anti-oxidant mineral selenium. Since selenium is part of the anti-oxidant enzyme glutathione peroxidase it may well help prevent the build up of arterial plaque by preventing damage to artery walls. Selenium is now widely available as a supplement in doses ranging from 30mcg to 100mcg. These doses are absolutely safe, but larger doses exceeding 1,000mcg should not be taken without the advice of your doctor or nutritionist since selenium does become toxic.

The minerals magnesium and calcium may both lower blood pressure through their effects on altering arterial tension. Of these, magnesium may be the most important for a healthy heart. In fact, some cardiologists believe that a significant proportion of heart attacks may occur not because of a blockage but because of coronary artery spasm, a cramp in the coronary arteries caused by magnesium deficiency. This discovery may explain why some angina patients do not experience angina pains on exertion or after heavy meals, but at times unrelated to fat intake.

Studies from Finland have shown that incidence of heart attacks are associated with areas low in magnesium and from animal studies it is known that a drop in magnesium concentration causes arteries to go into spasm. Magnesium is commonly deficient since it is mainly found in green leafy vegetables, nuts and seeds which are infrequently eaten by many people. It is also depleted rapidly by stress and by diuretic drugs, so frequently used to lower blood pressure.[37]

Although calcium deficiency can also raise blood pressure drinking lots of milk may not be advisable for those at risk from cardiovascular disease. Recent research is suggesting a link between coronary heart disease and milk consumption. Why this might be is not yet established. However most dietary sources of magnesium are also high in calcium.

The healthy heart plan

1. Avoid sugar, salt and too much saturated fat
These are the three main baddies, but too much unsaturated fat, especially if used in cooking, is bad too. So keep your overall fat intake down. How? Eat more vegetarian foods and substitute fish and chicken instead of meat. 50% to 75% of the calories in a steak are derived from fat, for skinless chicken its 30% and cod 8%. Have skimmed milk and less cheese. Don't have more than five eggs a week. They're 66% fat. Most 'fast' hamburger dishes have the equivalent of eight teaspoons of butter in them. If you crave salt you may be zinc deficient and need the salt to taste your food. Take a 15mg zinc supplement each day and leave out salt and salted foods for one month strictly. Salt is a pickler and you are the pickle. You really don't need it. Instead of sugar, chocolate, honey or large quantities of dried fruit have large quantities of fresh fruit instead.

2. Stop smoking
Smoking triggers off cell proliferation, starves healthy cells of oxygen, thickens the blood and raises your blood pressure. In fact, of the deaths caused by smoking twice as many are due to diseases of the heart and circulation than due to lung cancer. No wonder smokers increase their risk of a heart attack by 70%.

3. Keep fit and not fat
Even 30 minutes a week of aerobic exercise (raising your pulses to 80% of its maximum) is enough to maintain the fitness of your cardiovascular system. More strengthens your heart and arteries. It also helps to boost your metabolic rate and keep you slim. Being overweight puts an extra strain on the heart and arteries.

4. Avoid prolonged stress
Keep cool. Stress raises blood pressure by causing the blood vessels to constrict and the heart to beat fast. Notice your signs of tension (clenched fist, tight shoulders, nail biting, shallow breathing etc.) and see what circumstances make you stressed. Notice how you react. Do you drink more, eat more, become hyperactive, get cross? When you know what causes your stress and how you react you're half way there. The other half is dealing with these situations. Stimulants like coffee, tea, cola drinks and alcohol also cause similar harmful effects to your heart and arteries. Don't drink more than two glasses/cups a day of any of these.

5. Boost your anti-oxidant nutrients
Vitamin A, C, E and the minerals selenium, zinc and manganese all help to dispose of dangerous oxides that can damage arteries. Animals supplemented with these have a much reduced risk of heart disease. B vitamins area also important. B_3 helps to lower blood cholesterol and B_6 helps to metabolize fats.

The minerals potassium, calcium and magnesium all help to lower blood-pressure. Fruits are rich in potassium and green leafy vegetables are high in calcium and magnesium which are needed as well by the heart itself. All these need to be supplemented to ensure maximum protection.

6. Check your blood pressure and blood fats every three years
Blood pressure is a measure of the health of your arteries. Two figures are measured: the systolic

pressure, when the heart has just beaten and the pressure is greatest, and the diastolic pressure when the pressure is least in the lull between beats. Your blood-pressure is best maintained below 140/90. An even better predictor of your risk is a 'lipid profile'. This measures cholesterol, triglycerides and HDL in the blood. This can be arranged through your doctor.

CHAPTER 4.2

Nutrition and immune power

—OVERVIEW—

The world contains many different types of micro-organisms, many of which have the power to inflict great harm to us. Thus we have developed two lines of defence against attacking micro-organisms. The first line aims to stop them entering the body in the first place. The skin forms a germ-tight layer around the body restricting entry to cuts, and the natural orifices of the body (mouth, nose etc.) Acid in the stomach, which kills many micro-organisms entering with food; and cilia and mucus in the airways, which trap micro-organisms, both increase the effectiveness of this first line of defence.

Inevitably micro-organisms will enter and we need a second line of defence to deal with them. This is known as the immune system. This system is based both within the blood-stream and the lymphatic system. The main defenders within the immune system are white blood cells, and broadly speaking there are two major types. The first type (which includes macrophages and neutrophils) destroy micro-organisms by phago-cytosis. In this process the micro-organism is engulfed by the phagocytic cell and eaten up. Phagocytic cells form a general line of defence that kill anything foreign.

The second type of defenders are lymphocytes. These have the ability to recognize any particular breed of micro-organism, and then initiate a powerful attack geared to specifically destroying

that particular type by producing antibodies. There are two main types of lymphocyte, T-lym-phocytes and B-lymphocytes. Both T- and B-lymphocytes are not all the same. They contain many different variations each with the ability to recognize a particular type of micro-organism. Once a micro-organism is identified by the appropriate lymphocyte, the lymphocyte breeds and produces a whole army of clones designed specifically to destroy the particular micro-organisms.

In this way we develop immune power, the ability to fight off infections, like colds, flu and more serious viruses like AIDS. But sometimes the invader comes from within. Cells, when damaged, may become cancerous, which means they rapidly multiply. Just like a virus the immune system learns to recognize these aberrant cells and, if strong, destroys them before they can do harm.

The arrival of AIDS, now carried by over ten thousand people in Britain, has highlighted the importance of a strong immune system. But long before AIDS diseases of the immune system have rated highly in causes of suffering and even death. Cancer, pneumonia, flu, food poisoning and rheumatoid arthritis are just some of the diseases of the immune system. Many involve an initial insult, whether viral, bacterial, or in the case of cancer, exposure to carcinogens. But it is those with a weak immune system that suffer most.

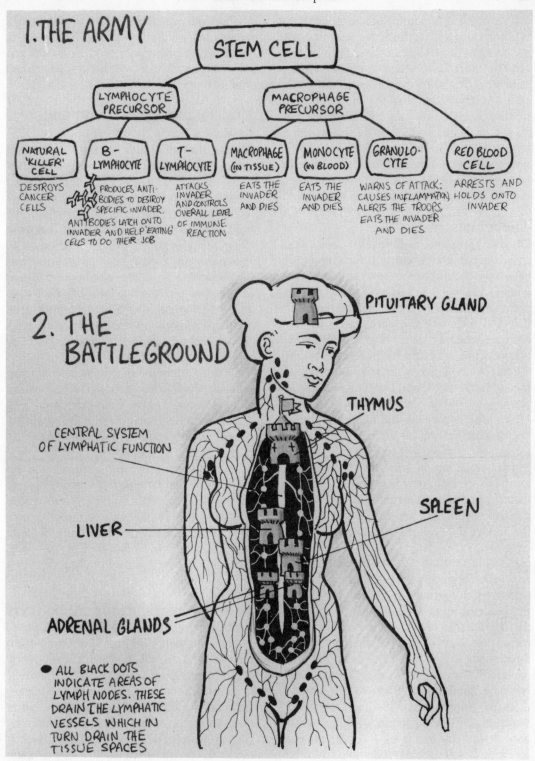

Figure 4.2.1 — *The immune system*

Over one billion pounds of research money is poured into finding drugs that will wipe out the invader. But perhaps we should be working out how to make ourselves strong rather than wiping out the enemy with drugs. Louis Pasteur said that it was the host, the human body's defence, not the invading organism that we should focus on. And ironically, the evidence suggests that, by feeding animals and ourselves with antibiotic and anti-viral agents the bacteria and viruses develop resistance, so new drugs have to be invented. It's a vicious circle.

The white army

Our body's defence against alien invaders is called the immune system. It consists of various cells called antibodies, macrophages and lymphocytes with a 'search and destroy' mission against defective cells, viruses and food particles that find their way uninvited inside us. For example, when we are exposed to a cold virus that we've had before, the B-lymphocytes release specific 'antibodies' designed to attach only to the 'antigen', which is the virus, and stop it attaching to our body cells and causing damage. Meanwhile, macrophages and T-lymphocytes are beckoned to the scene of the crime. These engulf the invader and begin to ingest and destroy it by releasing all sorts of chemicals. More than fifty chemicals secreted from macrophages have been identified so far. They also produce 'free radicals', dangerous forms of oxygen, which destroy the invader, but must themselves be destroyed once their job is over. This is done with anti-oxidants, like vitamins C and E and anti-oxidant enzymes, like glutathione peroxidase, which is dependent on selenium. As well as lymphocytes that boost the immune response there are those that stop the reaction and restore peace once the invasion is over. These are called suppressor T-lymphocytes.

And if that wasn't enough, there are additional components called NK (Natural Killer), lympho-cytes, the complement system and interferon, which all play a part in winning the battles that go on every day inside us. NK cells are our strongest ally against cancer cells. Interferon also suppresses cancer-cell growth.

And finally, when an infection is raging through our bodies, we develop a fever. This increases the activity of macrophages, and the levels of iron which the invader needs for survival are reduced in the blood.

Understanding auto-immune diseases

A weak immune system can result in frequent colds and infections. But more dangerous than this is an over-aggressive immune system that doesn't know when to stop reacting and what to react to. Food allergy is an example of the immune system over-reacting. More serious is rheumatoid arthritis, where antibodies to antibodies are produced. This is known as 'rheumatoid factor' and marks this form of joint inflammation as separate from other forms of arthritis. Diseases like SLE (systemic lupus erythematosus), where antibodies that attack normal healthy cells are produced, can often be deadly.

A strong immune system means a greater resistance both to infections and colds but also to auto-immune diseases, cancer and ageing. And there is no stronger way to fortify your immune system than through optimum nutrition.

The components of our white army are made primarily of protein and adequate protein nutrition is vital for a strong immune system. Protein deficiency has been shown to reduce lymphocyte and interferon production and to prevent the destruction of cancer cells. Since fat and cholesterol both weaken the immune system it is best to derive protein from lean meat or a vegetarian source.

The micronutrient immune boosters

B vitamin deficiency has long been known to affect immunity. People suffering from pantothenic acid or B_6 deficiency have atrophy of the thymus gland and spleen, which is where the basic material for lymphocytes and macrophages is made. Severe B_6 deficiency results in no antibody formation at all! Ideal intake for B_6 goes up with protein intake and doses well in excess of 100mg are often required for maximum immune power. The same is also true for pantothenic acid (B_5), where up to 2,000mg have been used. These B vitamins should always be taken with a B complex and mineral formula providing zinc and manganese.

Both folic acid and vitamin B_{12} are needed for proper production of lymphocytes, the white blood cells, as well as being vital for red blood-cell health and the transport of oxygen. But most important of all the vitamins is vitamin C. Despite some damning research of vitamin C's anti-cold properties, there is no doubt that vitamin C plays a key role in immunity. Animals deficient in vitamin C produce less T-lymphocytes, and when vitamin C is supplemented produce more. These white blood cells travel faster to the scene of the crime when vitamin C is present.

Vitamin C and the common cold

Recent research has also implicated vitamin C as a potent stimulant for interferon production. As an anti-oxidant it also helps mop up the free radicals, and is known to prevent nitrates and amines combining to produce the deadly car-cinogen, nitrosamine. Vitamin C has also been shown to wipe out the AIDS virus in laboratory experiments.[38]

Vitamin C's role in preventing colds may act primarily through immune boosting. However, immediate use of a megadose of vitamin C once a cold has started may also alter the pH balance of the blood, weakening the virus. Between 2,000 and 4,000mg of vitamin C is recommended on a daily basis, although 10,000mg a day is often needed to stop a cold or 'flu' that has already started.

Vitamin C's potency depends in part on the amount of vitamin E available. Also an anti-oxidant, vitamin E appears to be freed from its complex with the dangerous oxide radicals to fight another battle when high levels of vitamin C are also present. Vitamin E in turn protects vitamin A from oxidation. but most of all, large doses (800 to 1,600iu per day) have been shown to improve immune response, increasing B- and T-lymphocytes. In animals exposed to infection, vitamin E gives a four-fold increase in survival rate. The most active form of vitamin E is d-alpha tocopherol (not dl-alpha tocopherol) which is a natural source. Other tocopherols exist which may also have a role to play. Nuts and seeds provided mixed tocopherols. Make sure these are fresh to minimize the amount of rancid oils present.

Strengthening your resistance to infection

Before any virus or bacteria can do damage they must cross the first line of defence — your inside skin. This may be the lungs, or the intestinal tract. Either way, vitamin A strengthens these mem-branes against invaders. It also boosts production of virus-digesting enzymes and, when given in doses of 30,000 to 50,000iu to surgery patients, prevents the post-operative drop in lymphocyte counts which leaves the patient open to infection. No wonder high levels of vitamin A, particularly beta-carotene, are associated with very low risk of cancer.

But vitamin A itself can be toxic — at least in the animal form called retinol. Beta-carotene, the vegetable form found in orange-coloured foods including carrot, beetroot, apricots, peaches and green leafy vegetables, is quite safe in large doses. However, beta-carotene is one-sixth as potent as retinol in vitamin A activity and as the dose increases, less is converted to the active form by the liver. This mechanism is probably nature's way of preventing toxicity in animals eating large quantities of vitamin A rich fruits and vegetables.

The beta-carotene form of vitamin A has also been found to be an anti-oxidant at extremely low oxygen pressures found inside cells. Many studies show beta-carotene levels correlate better with low risk of certain cancers than do retinol levels.

The zinc — cold connection

'It is clear that zinc has a profound influence on immune responses' reports one of Britain's leading experts on nutrition and immunity, Dr Stephen Davies. 'When zinc is deficient, children become prone to infections.'[39] The thymus also atrophies, according to work by Dr Golden in Jamaica.[40] So pronounced is this effect that after only ten days of zinc supplementation at a level of 2mg per kg bodyweight, thymus size measurably increases. Another study reported a 221% increase in T-lymphocyte function once zinc deficiency had been corrected.

Zinc is probably the most deficient mineral in Britain. Our average intake is between 9 and 10mg, well short of the 15mg or more that we need. Stress depletes zinc, so does pregnancy, puberty and lactation. Zinc is needed to heal wounds and fight off infection. Vegetarians and anorexic patients are also at risk of zinc deficiency.

A recent study showed promising effects on reducing the duration of colds by sucking up to twelve lozenges containing 23mg of zinc.[41] This has given rise to a number of lozenges on the market, most containing little more than 5mg of zinc. Rheumatoid arthritis sufferers often have low zinc status and supplementing zinc decreases the inflammatory response.

Selenium and other essential elements

Copper, zinc and selenium are all involved in anti-oxidant enzyme reactions, but leader of the pack is definitely selenium. The anti-oxidant enzyme, glutathione peroxidase (GP) is so dependent on selenium that a ten-fold increase in selenium intake in the diet causes a two-fold increase in circulating GP. Low levels of selenium are associated with increased risk of cancer, cardiovascular disease and premature ageing. Selenium also works with vitamin E to boost antibody formation and lymphocyte production of the inflammatory agent, leukotrienes. If this is so, selenium should be beneficial for those with auto-immune diseases like rheumatoid arthritis.

In animal studies, selenium prevents the formation of cancer, preventing the cancer cells from dividing. Coeliac patients have a particularly high incidence of tumours and low levels of selenium.

High selenium intake is a wise precaution against cancer. Most of us get between 25 and 60mcg a day, and need anything from 50 to 200mcg for optimum immune function, so supplements are often necessary. But the form of selenium makes a difference. Selenomethionine, provided in selenium yeast, appears less effective, because these selenium amino acids

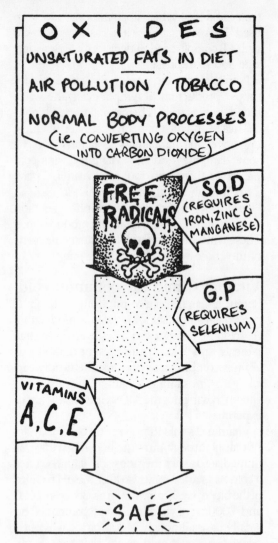

Figure 4.2.2 — *How anti-oxidants disarm oxides*

become integrated into cells and get broken down into organic compounds which are lost from the body. Sodium selenite is the preferred form by most selenium research. (Selenate seems favoured in New Zealand.)

Having looked at how the immune system works and which nutrients are needed to boost immune power let's consider the two most common immune diseases, cold and cancer.

Combating colds

Cold viruses are around us all the time. They

enter the body through food, drink or the air we breathe. They aren't actually alive but can take on life by invading and taking over the body cells. But normally theirs is a short life as our immune army swings rapidly into action.

Every minute of every day your body makes literally millions of special cells called lymphocytes, the troops of your immune defences. The first line of defence are the T-lymphocyte 'scout' cells. On sighting a cold virus they cling on tight and whistle up the rest of the troops. Among these are B-lymphocytes which produce tailor-made weapons, called antibodies, to the particular antigens. Within seconds your lymphocytes produce thousands of antibodies which tag onto the cold viruses and release deadly chemicals. If this wasn't enough already, along come the 'macrophages' which literally means 'big eaters'. These gobble up and digest any remaining infected cells.

If the battle has been long and hard you'll feel exhausted, blocked up, headachy, may be feverish and have swollen lymph nodes in the neck, groin and armpits, where the lymphocyte troops collect and bring infected cells for their final destruction.

The secret to stopping a cold before it starts is boosting your immune power. More and more research, mainly in the past four years, has confirmed that what you eat makes the biggest difference to immune strength. Vitamin C, A, E, B_6 and zinc are your strongest allies. Here are ten tips to kill a cold dead in its tracks.

1. Keep on guard

Even when there's no cold in sight it pays to keep your intake of vitamins A, C, E, B complex and the minerals zinc, calcium and magnesium high. Carrots, tomatoes, beetroot and apricots are good sources of A and so is fish. All fresh fruits and green peppers are rich in vitamin C and nuts and seeds are good sources of vitamin E. B complex vitamins are found in fresh fruit and vegetables and are higher in whole grains. Zinc is rich in all meat and fish and also wheatgerm and seeds. A basic multivitamin and mineral supplement containing 1,000mg of C 7,500iu of A and 7mg zinc is a good insurance policy.

2. Reinforce the troops when the risks are high

Your immune army becomes sluggish in cold weather and severely weakened by alcohol, cigarettes (and cannabis), high fat or protein deficient diets, stress and lack of sleep. So if you're burning the candle at both ends this is the time to boost your immune power by supplementing a further 2,000mg of C, 200mg of B_6 and 20mg of zinc. (Supplements exist which combine B_6 with zinc.)

3. Spot the early warning signs

Did you feel worse than usual this morning? Was it hard to get out of bed? Were your eyes bloodshot or did you feel a tickle in your throat? Did you sneeze or have to clear your throat or nose? Did you have watery or itchy eyes? These can all be signs of a cold getting started. If these coincide with a late night or if you've been in contact with someone with a cold this is the time to go into 'red alert' and use optimum nutrition to turn on full immune power, explained in the next seven points.

4. Saturate yourself with vitamin C

Countless studies have demonstrated vitamin C's cold fighting potential. As many more have shown unclear results. Why the difference? The difference is dose. When you take enough vitamin C to saturate the blood-stream cold viruses really suffer. For most people saturation is achieved with 2,000mg of C (two 1 gram tablets) every three hours. Some need less, some need more. If you get diarrhoea or stomach pain you need less. If this dose has no effect try taking more. As long as you drink plenty of liquids when taking this much vitamin C you could take four times this amount without harm.

5. Suck lo-zinc-ges

Zinc is the mighty mineral as far as immune power is concerned. In one study at the University of Texas sixty-five people suffering with a cold were given either zinc lozenges or a dummy lozenge to suck every two hours. After seven days 86% of those sucking zinc lozenges no longer had a cold, compared to less than half of those in the other group.[41] Zinc lozenges are widely available. Some unfortunately are full of sugar and contain little zinc. Go for those sweetened with fructose with at least 50mg of zinc gluconate in each tablet. This will give you 5mg of actual zinc and six or more of these in a day will give you a definite immune boost.

6. **Eat a mucus-free diet**
Some foods create mucus in the body. These include all fatty foods especially milk produce, eggs and red meat. This mucus clogs up the lymphatic vessels, along which your immune troops travel, making it harder for them to reach the scene of the crime. Fruits and vegetables are mucus-free.

7. **Keep drinking**
When under viral attack your immune system must get rid of toxic debris, which it does via the kidneys and bladder. This is why frequent urination is often a sign of infection. Drinking a lot helps the kidneys do their job. Drink water, herb teas, diluted fruit juice or vegetable juices, especially carrot which is high in vitamin A. Aim to drink about three pints of fluids a day.

8. **Keep the heat on**
Although being in a stuffy environment doesn't help, keeping warm does. The immune system works better when hot. That's what fevers are all about. Your body turning on the heat to boost your immune army.

9. **Keep cool**
You can prolong your cold by working too hard or exposing yourself to stressful situations. So keep cool and take it easy for a couple of day, then you'll be back in action faster.

10. **Think positive**
Your attitude can also make a difference. Dr Carl Simonton has, for over a decade, recorded better recovery from cancer, a far stronger opponent than the cold virus, in sufferers using positive guided imagery. So don't think 'Oh God, I feel awful'; imagine your immune army fighting hard and winning.

Cancer and nutrition
Cancer is the second most common cause of

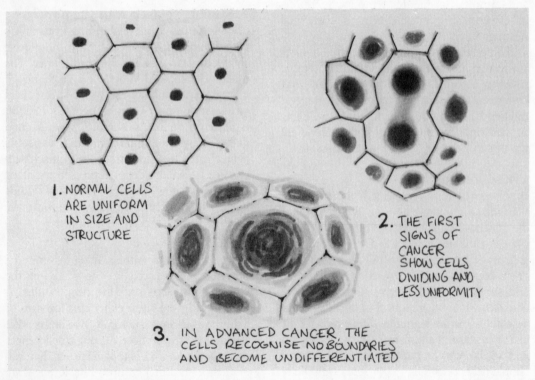

Figure 4.2.3 — *Normal cells* vs *cancer cells*

death in Britain. The incidence of certain types of cancer has dramatically increased this century due to greater exposure to cancer producing agent called carcinogens, and reduced ability to ward off cancer cells. Any body cell can become a cancer cell. When a cell is deprived of oxygen which it needs to produce energy it may revert to an earlier mechanism for deriving energy, not requiring energy. Like primitive cells, these cells grow rapidly then divide into two cells. Under the microscope these new cells lose regular shape and become undifferentiated, which means they fail to recognize the boundaries set by their neighbours. These are cancer cells and when the mass of cells is sufficiently large cancer may be diagnosed. When the primary tumour (cancer cell mass) is sufficiently large it enters a second phase called metastasis. Here small clusters of cells break off and cancer develops in other parts of the body. These are called secondary tumours.

Avoiding carcinogens

The initiation of a cancer cell depends on lack of oxygen, most commonly caused by cell damage, affecting either the behaviour of the cell or the permeability of the membrane of the cell. Substances which induce this damage are 'carcinogens'. The first line of defence is to avoid carcinogens. Benzopyrene from cigarettes, for example, is a powerful carcinogen which damages cells in the lungs. However, not all carcinogens are avoidable. In large enough amounts many common food dyes and preservatives are carcinogenic. So are many detergent, plastics and even radiation from the sun. However, it is possible and sensible to limit exposure to many of these substances.

One of the most potent carcinogens of all are peroxides, the by-products of breathing. We therefore have anti-oxidant enzymes to destroy these harmful oxides. Vitamins A, C and E are anti-oxidants, and the minerals selenium, copper, zinc and manganese are involved in anti-oxidant activity. Maintaining a strong anti-oxidant army is the second line of defence. But even so all of us do have some cancer cells and these need to be recognized as alien cells and destroyed and removed by our army of macrophages and lymphocytes, the immune system. So boosting immunity is the third line of defence against cancer.

There are three categories of cancer. Carcinomas are the most common and occur in epithelial cells that cover tissues and line body cavities. The most common carcinomas are breast, lung, colon and stomach. These are the most common forms of cancer and occur mainly in adults. Sarcomas are less common and more malignant. These occur in connective tissue — muscle, bone or cartilage. The third group, leukaemia, includes what we know as leukaemia which is an overproduction of white blood cells, followed by an under-production. Myelomas and lymphomas also fit into this category and affect bone marrow, from which all white blood cells are made. Leukaemias are more common in children.

The risk factors for cancer

There are many known risk factors for these different forms of cancer, most of which are easily avoided. The chart below shows which factors are associated with which form of cancer.

Lung cancer	Cigarettes (90% of victims smoke)
Colon cancer	Low fibre diet
Uterine cancer	Oestrogen (the pill)
Cervical cancer	Early sex with multiple partners
Esophageal cancer	Smoking and alcohol
Bladder cancer	Industrial carcinogens
Breast cancer	Oestrogens, excess dietary fat
Skin cancer	Overexposure to sun

Chart 4.2.1 — *Risk factors for cancer*

Treating cancer with optimum nutrition

The three methods used in the treatment of cancer are surgery, radiation and chemotherapy. Surgery aims to remove the cancer growth but does nothing to prevent a recurrence of a tumour. Radiation, while killing off cancer cells, also destroys some healthy cells and weakens the immune system even further. Depending on the length of treatment it often has pronounced side effects. Chemotherapy involves giving 'cytotoxic' drugs — substances that can kill cancer cells. Many cytotoxic agents also kill healthy cells as well as weakening the immune system. However a new generation of drugs that latch on to the cancer cells only are in the process of being developed and may provide a safer form of chemotherapy.

Nutrition can help combat cancer in many ways. First, some nutrients make cells strong enough to resist the initial onslaught, perhaps by a free oxidizing radical. Secondly, once the cancer cells are proliferating nutrients boost the immune system's ability to curb the growth. Thirdly, nutrition helps to protect neighbouring cells from free oxidizing radicals created by the cancer cells. And finally, and most controversially, some nutrients are thought to be cytotoxic agents themselves. In recent years three particular nutrients have stood out as potential anti-cancer agents. They are vitamin C, selenium and beta-carotene, the vegetarian form of vitamin A.

Vitamin C and cancer

Cancer patients have repeatedly been shown to have low levels of vitamin C in blood and body tissues. Those with higher blood levels have a better survival rate. One reason vitamin C may help is that it strengthens connective tissue, providing more resistance to the cancer for spreading. In 1969 Dr Burk, working at the National Cancer Institute, found vitamin C to have a cytotoxic effect on cancer cells. It also increases production of lymphocytes and can destroy some carcinogens like acetaldehyde and benzopyrenes found in cigarettes. Another common carcinogen, nitrosamines, are disarmed by vitamin C.

Although normal people supplementing 10 to 200mg a day have a lower risk of cancer, supplementing even 1,000mg appears to have little or no effect in raising blood levels in cancer patients. More is needed. One study by Linus Pauling and Dr Ewan Cameron gave 10,000mg of vitamin C a day to untreatable cancer patients which resulted in a survival rate four times longer than those not supplemented.[42] Similar results have been found in other studies throughout the world, but only when using at least 5,000mg or more a day.

Beta-carotene, vegetarian diets and cancer

Beta-carotene is a precursor for vitamin A. Vitamin A, C and E are all anti-oxidants. So it was assumed that when high levels of beta-carotene in the blood were found to indicate a low incidence of cancer it was because beta-carotene was converted into vitamin A. However it is now known that beta-carotene is an anti-oxidant in its own right and can function better in low oxygen environments (for example in and around cancer cells) than vitamin A, C or E. Many popular diets for cancer use large quantities of vegetable and carrot juice with good results. The high beta-carotene content of these juices is probably why.

However, another possible reason involving essential fatty acids, discovered from experimenting with vegetarian diets in animals with cancer, may also play a part. Linoleic acid, present in nuts, seeds and vegetable oils is converted into prostaglandin series 1 and 2. In reality very little prostaglandin series 2 is made. Cells need both types of prostaglandin and provided sufficient linoleic acid is provided by diet there is no problem. However, cancer cells in animals have proven to be particularly bad at converting linoleic acid into prostaglandin series 2. However milk products and meat provide another fatty acid called arachidonic acid, which can be directly converted in prostaglandin series 2. If this is the case, and the evidence is that it is, then vegan diets, free from meat or milk, would selectively starve cancer cells but not healthy cells of this vital component. In animal studies cancer masses do decrease far more rapidly on vegan diets. Whether the same is true for humans is not yet established.

Selenium protects against breast cancer

A link between selenium and cancer was first discovered in 1959 by Gerard Schrauzer.[44] He divided the USA into high, medium and low risk

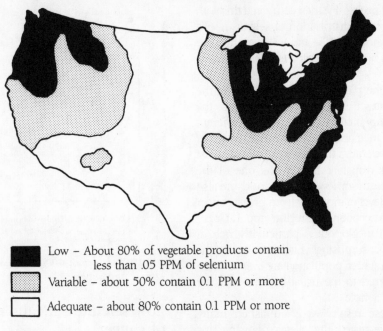

Low – About 80% of vegetable products contain less than .05 PPM of selenium

Variable – about 50% contain 0.1 PPM or more

Adequate – about 80% contain 0.1 PPM or more

Source: Data from USDA Technical Bulletin No. 758 (1967)

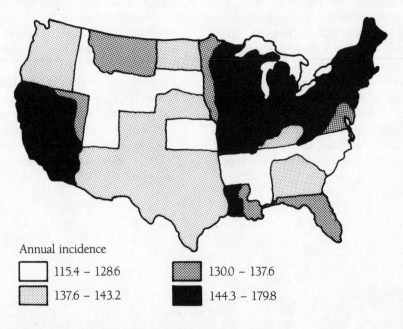

Annual incidence

115.4 – 128.6

130.0 – 137.6

137.6 – 143.2

144.3 – 179.8

Source: Schrauzer, G. 1959. *Bioinorganic Chemistry* 2(4)

Figure 4.2.4 – *Geographical distribution of cancer v selenium levels in the US*

cancer areas based on the incidence of cancer per 100,000 people. He then compared this with the geographical distribution of selenium. His results are shown below and indicate the clear relationship between cancer and selenium levels in the soil.

Later on, he plotted a graph comparing the mortality rates from breast cancer against the average dietary intake for twenty-seven different countries. Once again he found that the lower the level of selenium the higher the rate of breast cancer. Unfortunately, Britain has one of the lowest selenium soil levels in the world and also a very high level of mortality from breast cancer — with one exception. The region around Upper Sheringham in Norfolk is particularly rich in selenium. Not surprisingly, fifteen per cent of the Upper Sheringham population are over seventy-five, compared to the usual five per cent for Britain as a whole.

Since these results were published many studies have tested the effects of using this harmless mineral both to prevent and treat cancer in man and animals. So conclusive were the animal studies that most animal feeds are now enriched with selenium. For example, one study fed sodium selenite in drinking water to a strain of mice who were particularly susceptible to cancer. After fifteen months, 10% of these mice had developed cancer, compared to 82% in a similar group of mice not give selenium.

This sort of result has been so frequently duplicated that there is no doubt that selenium supplementation, or eating selenium-rich foods does prevent cancer in animals. But what about humans?

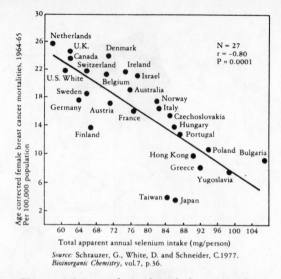

Source: Schrauzer, G., White, D. and Schneider, C.1977. *Bioinorganic Chemistry*, vol.7, p.36.

Figure 4.2.5 — *Relationship of selenium intake to cancer mortalities*

Low selenium means high risk of cancer

The positive effects of selenium may apply to us too. We know, from a number of research studies, that some people with cancer have lower than usual selenium levels in their blood. However, despite some promising results achieved using selenium on animals, virtually no studies have been carried on man using selenium supplementation. The National Research Council of the USA reported in 1982 that selenium may offer some protection against the risk of cancer, though the evidence is limited. They do not advise a greater supplement than 200mcg per day except with medical supervision.

CHAPTER 4.3

Overcoming food allergies

—OVERVIEW—

The term 'food allergy' is frequently used for almost any complaint connected with food, from indigestion to a psychological aversion to a particular food. So it's good to be clear what an allergy is, and how it differs from the broader concept of food intolerance. A food intolerance is any type of adverse reaction to a particular food. For instance, someone who does not produce enough bile will have difficulty digesting fats and react adversely to a high fat meal. However an allergy is a particular type of food intolerance that results in an immune response. The allergen, when absorbed by the gut, is regarded as an alien invader just like a virus or strain of bacteria, and attacked by the immune system.

The symptoms of an allergy vary from individual to individual and can literally encompass the whole body. They can include physical symptoms, like dark circles under the eyes, digestive complaints, mental and behavioural problems ranging from depression through to hyperactivity and aggressive behaviour, general feelings of fatigue and illness, and finally specific diseases like rheumatoid arthritis. In most cases, symptoms become chronic and remain with the sufferer most of the time. Obviously all of these conditions can be brought on for other reasons making diagnosis particularly important. People who are allergic are more likely to be allergic to their favourite foods or foods they eat on a daily basis since an allergy is akin to an addiction.

The most valid way of testing for an allergy is by means of an exclusion diet. Suspected foods are eliminated for a period of ten to thirty days and then reintroduced to the diet. During the beginning of an exclusion diet a withdrawal reaction is very often encountered with symptoms getting much worse. This is followed by a period of considerable improvement often with symptoms disappearing altogether. However on reintroduction the symptoms return suddenly and dramatically making diagnosis possible. A number of laboratory tests are also available and are useful for people who cannot follow an exclusion diet.

One man's food is another man's poison — so the saying goes, which illustrates how individual reaction to ordinary foods have been around since the beginning. But only in the last ten years has the concept of food allergy become accepted by the medical profession.

What is an allergy?

An allergy is not the same as an adverse reaction to a substance. Many substances act as poisons, stimulants or irritants and may cause adverse reactions. These, if more pronounced in some people than others, are broadly referred to as intolerances. So someone without the enzyme, lactase, that breaks down lactose, is called lactose intolerant.

An allergy is different and is best understood

by explaining the mechanism that causes an allergy. As well as being equipped with an immune system designed to protect us from foreign bodies (whether foods, viruses or bacteria) we are also equipped with an immune system designed for tolerance. After all, if we reacted to any ingested substance life would be one permanent allergic reaction. It is the balance between tolerance and immunity that is at the core of allergy.

For example, the most important control of the allergic state is carried out by one variety of immune cell called the T-lymphocyte. There are two important varieties: the T 'helper' cell, which passes on instructions for antibodies to be made; and the T 'suppressor' cell, which is specifically sensitized to a particular allergen (the substance that causes the allergic reaction) and has the ability to switch off the activities of other cells which are programmed to mount an allergic response.

The balance between these two types of T-lymphocytes is controlled partly by the amount of the allergen and partly by nutrition and hormonal activity. For instance, the hormone thymosin is zinc dependent. When zinc supply is good and thymosin levels are high, more T suppressor cells are released, decreasing or eliminating the allergic response. Other factors, like stress, decrease the production of T-lymphocytes, which survive for about three months.

With this model in mind it is easy to see why proper nutrition decreases allergic response; why smaller amounts of the allergen will mean a smaller reaction; why ingestion of a food that has been avoided for three months often causes no reaction although subsequent ingestion will — because the immune system has been primed; and why four day rotation diets or desensitization techniques may work by promoting tolerance through stimulation of T suppressor cells.

The most common allergies

Knowing how allergic reactions occur does not, however, explain why they occur. Food allergies most commonly occur to staple foods, such as wheat, eggs and milk. Different hypotheses have been put forward to explain why these foods are more likely to offend. Grains, say some, are a recent addition to diet and we may not yet all have adapted to these foods. Milk is designed for baby mammals and not for adult humans. Others argue that it is the deterioration of our immune strength, through faulty diet and exposure to environmental toxins, that has led to the increasing incidence of allergy. Whatever the reason, most food allergies are to proteins within food, and similar proteins found within food families often cause an allergic reaction also. For example, someone allergic to milk is likely to react to cheese, less likely to react to yogurt where the protein has been somewhat altered, and is unlikely to react to butter which contains virtually no protein, just fat. The chart below shows the most common food and inhalant allergens, the group to which they belong and other members of the group.

Allergen	Group	Other group members	Allergen	Group	Other group members
Wheat	Grain	Rye, oats, barley	Oranges	Citrus fruit	Lemons, grapefruits
Milk	Dairy	Yogurt, cheese, butter	Yeast	Yeast	Bakers yeast
Eggs	Poultry	Chicken	Onions, garlic	Onions, garlic	Onions, garlic
Coffee	Pip, nut	Any nut or pip-containing fruit	Shellfish	Shellfish	Mussels, oysters, clams etc
Chocolate	Pip, nut	Any nut or pip-containing fruit	Crustaceans	Crustaceans	Crabs, lobsters, prawns
Nuts	Pip, nut	Any nut or pip-containing fruit	Certain colourings	Azo dyes	E100s (not all cause reactions)

Allergen	Group	Other group members	Allerge	Group	Other group members
Plums, strawberries	Salicylates	All berries, apricots, cherries, apples, raisins currants, prunes, almonds	Hair	Hair	Cats, dogs, horses
			Pollen	Grasses	
			Feathers		
Inhalants			Fumes	Hydro-carbons	Gas, diesel, petrol, cigarettes
House dust		House dust mite			

Chart 4.3.1 — *The most common allergens*

The symptoms and degree of allergic reaction vary from individual to individual and it is likely that a large proportion of the population have mild allergies. The most pronounced symptoms include eczema, asthma, rhinitis, perpetual 'colds', abdominal bloating, marked hyperactivity and irritable bowel problems. But other less obvious physical and psychological symptoms can be caused by allergic reactions. These include puffy face, puffy eyes, dark circles around the eyes, nasal drip or irritation, skin reactions, headaches, obesity, depression, mental confusion and forgetfulness, sleepiness, emotional instability and PMT symptoms.

Testing for allergens
Since having an allergy is somewhat akin to an addiction it is possible, and probable, that an individual is consuming unwittingly the substance they react to almost on a daily basis. This often causes symptoms to be mild and continuous, making it hard to detect what is causing the allergic reaction by observation. By avoiding the allergen symptoms improve so much that when the allergen is introduced in sufficiently large amounts the symptoms become clearly noticeable. This pattern is exploited in elimination diets.

Elimination diets
The simplest (in principle, not in practice) type of elimination diet is to fast on water for three to five days. Provided the person is healthy to start with this is not dangerous. However, it isn't easy and some allergists recommend eating only lamb and pears, or any other two foods unlikely to cause a reaction. An even easier approach is the 'caveman' diet which restricts the client to 'caveman' foods — meat, fish, vegetables and fruits. No grains, milk, sugar, alcohol, additives, chocolate, tea or coffee. Perhaps the most practical is to restrict the consumption of suspected foods only for a period of ten or more days. However, the latter two methods do depend on the client or nutritionist having a strong suspicion as to the likely offender. The most likely offending foods are those in the list above, that are eaten nearly every day and that the client would have difficulty in giving up.

The pulse test
The purpose of all these elimination diets is to return the person to a point of no reaction and improved health. If no change occurs in symptoms within a month of avoidance of foods, then it is unlikely that they have an allergy, or the appropriate foods have not yet been withdrawn. If symptoms have improved then likely allergens can be tested by reintroducing them one at a time into the diet on a daily basis. The pulse rate often increases noticeably after eating an allergen so, on first eating the food the pulse, recorded over one hour, can serve as a guide to potential allergic reactions.

Skin testing
Two methods exist for testing allergies by measuring the reaction on the skin. One involves scratching the skin, then introducing potential allergens to the scratch. If a reaction occurs a red inflamed area appears around the scratch within ten minutes, signalling an immune response. Scratch testing is most useful for allergic reactions that involve the skin or for inhalant allergens, but often fail to detect food allergens. More than one substance is tested at the same time.

The second method, intradermal testing, involves injecting small amounts of the potential allergen in solution under the skin. This produces a small bubble which again becomes inflamed within ten minutes if the reaction is positive. One of the drawbacks with this method is the length of time it takes to test many different substances.

Cytotoxic testing

Cytotoxic testing involves introducing potential allergens in solution to leucocytes (white blood cells) separated from whole blood. In this way fifty or more substances can be tested from one blood sample. If the leucocytes rupture or show other signs of reaction to the allergen the reaction is said to be positive. This method is particularly useful when there are clear signs of allergy but no clues as to what might be causing the problem.

Unfortunately, all methods of testing have their limitations, and probably the most accurate way of determining an allergen is avoiding the substance and then reintroducing it and observing the reaction.

Decreasing your allergic potential

Once allergens have been identified there are a number of ways of 'desensitizing' the individual. Firstly, the food can be avoided altogether. This is not always practical. The second method involves 'rotating' foods. This means that the allergen is only eaten every four or five days, which is thought to stimulate T lymphocyte suppressor cells. For example, if a person reacts to wheat, milk and nuts, then wheat could be eaten on Monday and Friday, milk on Tuesday and Saturday, and nuts on Wednesday and Sunday.

Desensitizing drops or injections can also be given to stimulate tolerance to the food. For many allergens there is a dose at which no reaction occurs, which can be determined by intradermal injections. The dose injected is diluted and diluted until no reaction occurs, then that dilution is given as drops or injection to encourage the development of tolerance to the allergen.

During any desensitization treatment it is wise to follow general guidelines for good nutrition and to ensure adequate supplementation of vitamin C, B_6, zinc and calcium, all of which help to reduce allergic response. When in the grips of an allergic reaction large amounts of vitamin C, B_6, B_5 or calcium are often helpful in stopping or reducing the reaction.

CHAPTER 4.4

Nutrition, the mind and behaviour

—OVERVIEW—

It is fairly easy to accept that sub-optimum nutrition can result in a whole variety of symptoms, particularly later in life. However for many people it is much harder to accept that nutrition can have a profound influence on the mind and behaviour. The first effects of sub-optimum nutrition are on behaviour since the brain is more sensitive than any other organ to small changes in nutrient supply from the diet. There are five main nutritionally related factors that can adversely influence behaviour.

The first is low blood sugar. This occurs following an over production of insulin in response to an adrenal stimulant or an excess of refined carbohydrates (see chapter 4.6). Although low blood sugar usually results in a loss of energy, it also increases aggressive tendencies and there seems to be a critical range for low blood sugar where there is sufficient energy for this to manifest itself in violent behaviour.

The second factor is lead toxicity. Lead is a brain poison that adversely effects intelligence, learning and general mental functioning. Its effects are particularly severe with children for whom lead can cross the blood brain barrier more easily, and is more readily retained.

The third factor is an allergy either to a particular food itself or to a chemical additive found in food. A food allergy can have a profound effect on behaviour particularly in children, and

often this is expressed as aggressive behaviour.

The fourth factor is alcoholism and drug addiction in general. At first sight this may not seem to be connected with nutrition at all. However researchers have found that just about all alcoholics have a very poor nutritional status as they obtain calories from alcohol, which is devoid of essential nutrients.

The fifth factor is an over or underproduction of histamine. Many schizophrenics have been found to have abnormal levels of the neuro-transmitter histamine. Excessive intake of copper lowers histamine and can result in disturbed behaviour. On the other hand excessive histamine production, which is an inherited trait, increases susceptibility to depression.

All of these factors can be helped through optimum nutrition.

Much can be learnt from old housewives, and the tale about fish being good for the brain is no exception. Our brains, like our bodies, need food of a special kind. Scientists are only beginning to unravel the complexity of our 3lbs of delicate software. Computer experts have estimated that it would take a computer the size of Buckingham Palace to hold the 15 trillion specific memories stored over a lifetime, and to carry out the complex calculations we call thinking. Our brain consists of many millions of nerve cells each cross-connected to each other by around 10,000 tentacle like connectors called dendrites. The electrical messages that pass between these cells are our thought processes, causing minute chemical changes in the levels of neuro (nerve) transmitter substances. One of these substances, acetylcholine, is made from the nutrient choline, particularly high in fish. The 'acetyl' part can only be made when enough vitamin B_5 (pantothenic acid) is present in our diets.

Natural tranquillizers

Another neurotransmitter, 'serotonin', helps to put you to sleep at night — and keeps you happy in the daytime. Serotonin is made from vitamin B_3 and the protein constituent, trytophan, provided there is enough B_6 present. Trytophan is now being used as a safe and non-addictive anti-depressant and sleep promoter. The

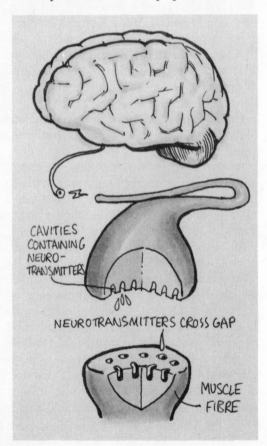

Figure 4.4.1 — *How neurotransmitters control nerve impulses*

minerals calcium and magnesium also act as natural tranquillizers. Calcium in particular is vital for proper nerve function and deficiency of calcium or magnesium can result in disturbed sleep and anxiety. Doses of at least 100mg B_6, 600mg calcium and 300mg of magnesium are usually needed to produce a result. Trytophan takes up to an hour to work, so should be taken in doses of one to four 500mg tablets, an hour before intended 'departure time' without food.

The sugar blues

But feeding the grey matter isn't just a matter of providing the right nutrients. It's also a question of balance. And the balance of the brain's most important nutrient, glucose, is the most delicate of all. A well balanced diet should consist of 60% of the energy as carbohydrates. Grains, nuts, seeds and vegetables provide complex carbohydrates. Fruit and, of course, sugar provide simple carbohydrates. 30% of all the energy we produce from these foods goes to power the brain. Equally important though are the micro-nutrients, the vitamins and minerals found in unrefined foods that act as catalysts in the many stages that turn the sugar you eat into energy. The most important nutrients are the minerals chromium, zinc, calcium and magnesium, and the vitamins B_1, B_2, B_3, B_5 and B_6 as well as vitamin C. These are often supplied in whole foods like wholegrains and vegetables, but can be almost completely lacking in refined foods. For example, the refining of sugar removes 95% of the chromium, refining flour removes 98% of the chromium and 78% of the zinc. By the age of fifty most people are severely deficient in chromium.

Ironically, frequent eating of refined carbohydrates like sugar or cakes, biscuits and even honey or excess dried fruit, can starve the brain of vital glucose. This happens because the body overreacts to the sudden increase in blood sugar levels by releasing too much insulin, causing a too sudden or too low drop in blood sugar. This can happen within twenty minutes or three hours of eating and leads to symptoms of confusion, forgetfulness, difficulty concentrating and 'blank' mind. And when these 'sugar blues' strike we soon unconsciously learn that the way to avoid these withdrawal effects, at least temporarily, is to have more. It's like an addiction. Too much of any stimulant, including tea or coffee can have the same effect because they cause the liver to mobilize sugar stores again raising blood sugar level.

Brain allergies

Dr Len McEwen, one of London's leading allergy researchers, believes that 'brain fag' caused by hypoglycaemia (low blood sugar levels) is a common symptom of food allergy.

> Many patients with what we call Allergic Psychological Syndrome, or APS, respond abnormally when given glucose by mouth. Three hours after the dose, when the blood sugar level should be returning to normal the APS sufferer's does not. It keeps dropping into the third and fourth hour. Sometimes the patient feels weak, shaky and sweaty. The symptoms can be relieved by more food.

One of the most common foods that this type of allergy sufferer often reacts to is grains and particularly wheat. One of the clues for allergy is craving for a particular food. Often the food that's hardest to give up is the likely offender. If you suspect you may be allergic to something, one simple test is to avoid any suspected foods for ten days and see what happens. If symptoms get worse for the first few days then food allergy should be suspected. However, if you have multiple food allergies, avoiding one food only may make little overall difference.

Mental illness — the histamine connection

Most food allergies involve the release of the hormone and neurotransmitter, histamine. This causes inflammatory reactions, for example the swelling and itching following an insect bite. Some individuals naturally produce large amounts of histamine. They are more prone to headaches, cold-like symptoms and allergies. A large proportion of schizophrenics are high in histamine. This imbalance makes them prone to severe depression and compulsive behaviour. Since histamine speeds up metabolism these people are rarely overweight, often hyperactive and are less hairy individuals with long toes and fingers and prominent veins — all methods of cooling down since fast metabolizers produce more heat.

These discoveries, pioneered by Dr Carl Pfeiffer, of the Brain Bio Center in New Jersey USA,[45] led to the discovery that anti-histamine nutrients vitamin C, calcium and the amino acid methionine could help to restore mental stability by balancing histamine levels.

Histamine, copper and mental illness

Histamine is not only a problem when levels are too high. Low levels, called histapenia, also upset brain chemistry. A larger proportion, about 50% of those with schizophrenia, are, according to Dr Pfeiffer, likely to be low in histamine. Histapenic patients tend to suffer from paranoia or hallucinations and are suspicious by nature.

The primary cause for low histamine is thought to be an accumulation of copper. This essential, but potentially toxic mineral has become increasingly available though its widespread use in water pipes. It is a strong antagonist to zinc and individuals low in zinc are therefore more susceptible to copper toxicity. Supplementing zinc and vitamin C helps to lower copper, while large amounts of B_3, B_{12} and folic acid have been shown to help raise histamine levels.

Deficiency of zinc and B_6 is another common cause for mental illness. This can result in the presence of kryptopyrroles in the urine (known as pyroluria) — an undesirable chemical complex that removes zinc and B_6 from the body. Kryptopyrroles were first discovered in the urine of schizophrenics in the 1950s, although it was then known as the 'mauve' factor, because when reacted with a reagent it turned mauve, and was not identified as kryptopyrrole for many years. The symptoms of pyroluria include depression, mental confusion, aggressive behaviour, white marks on the nails, pale skin, lack of dream recall, poor resistance to infection and a poor sense of taste. Treatment with large amounts of zinc (20 to 50mg daily) and B_6 (up to 500mg) lowers kryptopyrroles and reduces these symptoms.

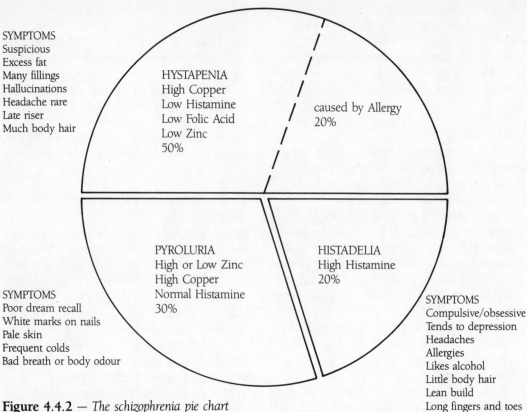

SYMPTOMS
Suspicious
Excess fat
Many fillings
Hallucinations
Headache rare
Late riser
Much body hair

HYSTAPENIA
High Copper
Low Histamine
Low Folic Acid
Low Zinc
50%

caused by Allergy
20%

PYROLURIA
High or Low Zinc
High Copper
Normal Histamine
30%

HISTADELIA
High Histamine
20%

SYMPTOMS
Poor dream recall
White marks on nails
Pale skin
Frequent colds
Bad breath or body odour

SYMPTOMS
Compulsive/obsessive
Tends to depression
Headaches
Allergies
Likes alcohol
Little body hair
Lean build
Long fingers and toes

Figure 4.4.2 — *The schizophrenia pie chart*

Alcoholism and addiction

Addiction to alcohol, heroin or other drugs has much in common with nutritional imbalances. High histamine types are particularly fond of alcohol and can usually tolerate it well. A large proportion of alcoholics are high histamine producers (histadelics). They use it as a 'slow suicide'. The belligerent, binge drinker is more likely to be low in histamine. Closely related to alcohol, many hypoglycaemics become addicted to alcohol instead of sugar. It is a common practice for alcoholics, when off drink, to consume large quantities of sugar in its place. Some drinkers are allergic to a component within the drink. This could be yeast, hops, barley or some other ingredient.

Identifying which of these factors plays a part in the addiction provides an important clue as to how to alter nutrition to reduce cravings. Work by Dr Stanley Schachter at New York's Columbia University has also shown that eating an alkaline diet reduces cravings for alcohol and cigarettes. Of course, large consumption of any of these drugs leads to nutritional deficiences which perpetuate the symptoms, so overall optimum nutrition is also important for reducing symptoms and craving.

Brain pollution

Like our environment, our brains are also subject to pollution. When you consider that we consume one gallon of pesticides and herbicides, thirteen pounds of additives and preservatives and breathe in one gram of toxic metals like lead each year it would be surprising if this didn't have an effect on our mental performance.

For the past six years, Professor Bryce-Smith from Reading University has been analysing mineral levels in placentas to work out just how important levels of toxic minerals are to mental development later in life. His results have confirmed the importance of low level lead for high level intelligence. He found that the higher the level of lead or cadmium in the mother's placenta the greater the risk of mental retardation in the child. Meanwhile in America, child psychiatrist Dr Needleman, has recently shown that lead levels at birth correlate with intelligence at age three.[12] One of the most worrying findings in these recent experiments is that there appears to be no 'safe' threshold for lead. These effects on intelligence occur, albeit to a lesser degree, at levels even below the average for children in Britain.

Lead affects brain power in many ways. During childhood, when mental development is most active, each nerve cell sends out about 10,000 connectors. These cross-connect with other nerve cells creating a network of awesome complexity. However, when lead levels in the brain are high a 10% reduction on cross-connections can occur. Lead also interferes with the electrical signal that passes between cells. Much like an out of tune car, lead causes the cell to misfire. In children this often results in symptoms of hyperactivity, disturbed sleep, emotional and aggressive outbursts, poor attention and slow learning. For adults symptoms include poor memory, mental confusion, head-aches and excessive sleepiness. Chemically, lead interferes with the action of essential minerals zinc and calcium. As well as avoiding potential sources of lead, Professor Bryce-Smith thinks we should be supplementing extra zinc and calcium, as well as eating foods high in these nutrients.

Another brain pollutant is aluminium. Found in large quantities in the brains of people suffering from senile dementia, aluminium was proposed in the seventies to be a 'memory blocker'. In 1986 a Medical Research Council confirmed that sufferers of Alzheimer's disease, a form of senile dementia, have unusual clusters of nerve cells in the brain which are saturated with aluminium. The widespread use of aluminium in pots and pans, food packaging, and even in antacids has led to increasingly high levels in man, where it

Food for thought		Brain nutrients (daily)	
Fish—	herring	Vitamin B$_1$ (thiamine)	100mg
	mackerel	Vitamin B$_2$ (riboflavin)	100mg
	salmon	Vitamin B$_3$ (niacin)	200mg
Egg yolks		Vitamin B$_5$ (pantothenate)	500g
Seeds —	sesame	Vitamin B$_6$ (pyridoxine)	200mg
	sunflower	Vitamin B$_{12}$ (cobalamin)	20mcg
Wholegrains —	rye	Folic acid	200mcg
	oats	Choline	500mg
	barley	Vitamin C	1,000mg
	rice	Zinc	15mg
Vegetables —	all especially green	Chromium	10mcg
	leafy vegetables	Calcium	175mg
	peppers	Magnesium	100mg
Fruits —	tropical fruits		
	mangoes		
	kiwis		
Oils —	cold-pressed		
	vegetable oil		
	1 tbspn a day		

Chart 4.4.2 — *Brain boosting nutrients*

accumulates since it is hard to get out of the body. There is some evidence that vitamin C and magnesium may help to reduce aluminium levels in the body.

Essential fatty acids and the brain

You might be surprised to learn that 30% of the brain is fat and that nearly a fifth of this is cholesterol. Just like electrical wires, nerves need to be insulated to stop short-circuiting. Special fats provide this insulation and the source of these fats is our diet. The essential fats, alpha-linolenic and linoleic acid, found in vegetable and seed oils, are in turn converted into more and more complex fats to be incorporated into nerve cells. Sometimes this conversion process isn't too efficient. In rare diseases, like multiple sclerosis, this conversion breaks down and the protective myelin sheath of the nerve degenerates, causing loss of muscle function and mental ability. Two types of fat found in nature are able to bypass some of these faulty conversion processes, making the body's job easier. One is gamma-linolenic acid from the evening primrose plant, the other is eicosapentaenoic acid (EPA for short!) found in oily fish. Although research into these oils is in its infancy they are both likely to be beneficial brain nutrients.

CHAPTER 4.5

Nutrition and arthritis

—OVERVIEW—

Although not as deadly as heart disease or cancer, arthritis is the most common form of degenerative disease. The American National Institute for Health, using X-ray analysis, estimates that 97% of the population over 60 years of age have arthritis.

Broadly speaking there are two different types of arthritis that both result in joint pain and inflammation, yet have completely different mechanisms and causes.

In osteoarthritis degeneration begins with the joint itself and is usually triggered by a calcium deficiency within the bones or a previous physical injury. The disease spreads outward causing inflammation in the surrounding area. Critical to this condition is maintaining proper calcium balance. This is regulated by calcium, magnesium and vitamin D intake together with proper thyroid and parathyroid function. Exercise also improves calcium balance, while obesity, bad posture and hard physical labour may contribute to the problem by putting further stress on weight bearing joints, which are prone to degeneration.

Rheumatoid arthritis is not a disease of the skeletal structure like osteoarthritis, but is a disease of the immune system, known as an auto-immune disease. Within the immune system are lymphocytes which are designed to track down any outside invaders and destroy them. In the case of an auto-immune disease they identify parts of the body as foreign and attack it by mistake. In rheumatoid arthritis it is the joints that are attacked. A number of different theories exist to explain this disease, however it is hard to treat and nobody has the complete answer. Allergies are often involved, and hormonal and prostaglandin imbalances may make the inflammation worse. Excesses of the minerals copper and iron, and deficiencies of zinc or manganese also exacerbate the problem and suggest a role of free radicals and oxidation in this disease.

The word arthritis means inflammation (itis) of the joint (arthron). There are many kinds of arthritis, some of which, contrary to this definition, result in calcium deposits in muscles. Most, but not all, have in common the misuse of calcium. (One exception is gout which causes pain usually in the feet and finger joints due to a build up of uric acid crystals.) In osteoarthritis joints degenerate. In rheumatoid arthritis joints can fuse together and distorted build ups of calcium cause enlarged joints. Many people suffer from degeneration of the vertebrae of the spine, usually suffering from backache and lack of flexibility. Only when the degeneration becomes pronounced does inflammation occur, and hence arthritis is diagnosed. Even more common is osteoporosis (porous bones), present particularly in women over fifty. This can lead to easy fracture. Underlying all these diseases is misuse of calcium.

Understanding calcium balance

Calcium is the most abundant mineral in the body, accounting for 1.6% of our body mass. Of the 1200 grams of calcium in us more than 99% are in the bones and teeth. The rest is present in muscles, nerves and the blood-stream where it plays a crucial role in many enzymes and the production of nerve signals and muscular energy.

Calcium is relatively well absorbed, with on average 30% of ingested calcium reaching the blood-stream. But its absorption into the blood-stream depends upon many factors. An excess of alcohol, a lack of hydrochloric acid, or an excess of acid forming foods (mainly protein) decrease its absorption. So does the presence of lead which competes for absorption sites. A

hormone produced by the parathyroid gland also helps absorb calcium. It does this by converting vitamin D into another hormone which makes the gut wall more permeable to calcium. So lack of vitamin D is another factor to consider. Parathormone also helps to keep calcium in circulation once absorbed, by reducing excretion of calcium via the kidneys.

Once in the body there are many factors which influence calcium balance. Once again, heavy metals like lead compete with calcium. So does sodium, tea, cocoa and red wine. In post-menopausal women the low levels of oestrogen also make calcium less retainable. One of the greatest factors is exercise or rather, lack of it. Studies by NASA, who had discovered losses of

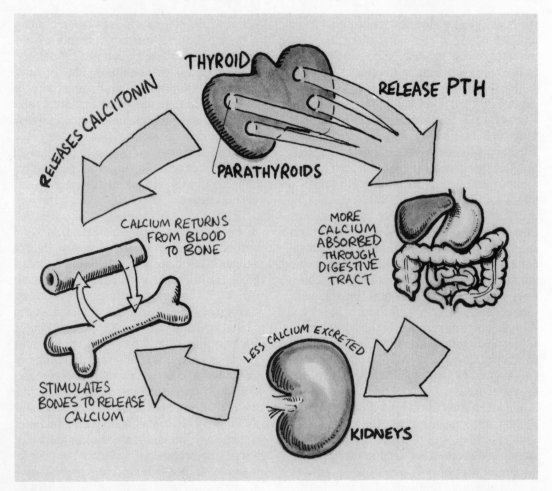

Figure 4.5.1 — *Calcium balance*

calcium in astronauts in zero gravity, showed that weight bearing exercise, for example walking, would raise calcium levels in the body by 2% or more.[46]

Once in the body calcium is constantly moving from blood to bone. Its release into the blood occurs when it is needed to stimulate muscles or nerves. Once this reaction is over the thyroid gland recalls calcium to the bones by secreting the hormone, calcitonin. An imbalance in the thyroid or parathyroid gland can also interfere with calcium balance.

Osteoarthritis

Osteoarthritis occurs through the gradual loss of calcium in joints, leading to their degeneration. This causes rough edges at the joints which may be audible and usually cause pain by inflaming the joint. With this loss of calcium from joints may also occur deposition of calcium in the wrong places, such as old injury sites and even in artery walls. These problems are not, however, a result of excess calcium but more the result of misuse and often deficiency of calcium.

One of the commonest causes for calcium imbalances is sugar and the overuse of stimulants, discussed in the next chapter. It is well known that diabetics and people with glucose intolerance have impaired calcium metabolism. So reducing sugar consumption and the use of stimulants is a vital part of the nutritional treatment of osteoarthritis.

But calcium deficiency, whether through poor absorption or insufficient diet is almost epidemic. The problem is most serious in post-menopausal women who suffer from demineralization of the bones earlier than men due to low circulating levels of oestrogen.

Osteoporosis

But for every one woman with post-menopausal arthritis many more have osteoporosis. A similar disease can occur due to the lack of vitamin D. This is called rickets in children and osteomalacia in adults and is different to osteoporosis in that the bones, instead of becoming porous and more brittle, become pliable often resulting in bow legs and bent fingers and toes.

Some research has indicated that, to maintain normal bone density in a post-menopausal woman 1,200 to 1,400mg of calcium must be ingested, and recent useful studies show that even 2,000mg only lightly slowed bone loss. Yet one survey in 1986 showed that 73% of women do not even get 500mg of calcium.

The stress connection

The dramatically increased need for calcium in

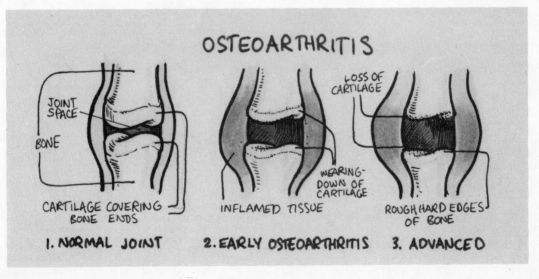

Figure 4.5.2 — *Osteoarthritis*

later years is not seen in primitive communities not eating the typical western diet. One likely probability is that the whole endocrine system gradually becomes inefficient through its over-stimulation from stress, sugar, coffee, tea, chocolate, alcohol and smoking. These factors also cause an even more significant loss of magnesium, which together with calcium, controls nerve and muscle cell reactions. Most of the calcium is extra-cellular, for example in the synapse, the gap between cells. In fact, the extracellular calcium level is some 10,000 times greater than inside the cell. To pass a nerve signal from one cell to another calcium ions are absorbed into the cell, then pumped out again. Most of the magnesium is within cells. A lack of magnesium leads to an increased intra-cellular calcium level which can cause cells to die.

The western diet, with a relatively large consumption of dairy produce is likely to provide relatively more calcium than magnesium, since dairy produce contains virtually no magnesium. Green leafy vegetables, nuts and seeds, as well as whole grains, contain significant amounts of both calcium and magnesium. These foods together with a moderate intake of dairy produce are the best way of getting as much calcium and magnesium as possible from the diet.

In the winter, calcium intake is particularly critical, because the presence of sunlight acting on the skin, converts chemicals in the body into vitamin D, which then aids the absorption of calcium. This conversion process is particularly active in autumn. So getting outdoors in the winter may help calcium balance.

However, supplements are needed, especially in the elderly to minimize the risk of arthritis. It is best to get three parts of calcium to two parts of magnesium. This ratio is often provided in dolomite tablets. Depending on other factors an overall intake of at least 750mg of calcium is recommended. Since diet provides 400 to 500mg an additional 250mg or more should be supplemented.

Rheumatoid arthritis

Rheumatoid arthritis, although having much in common with osteoarthritis, is very different in origin. It is usually caused by a faulty immune system which produces antibodies to its own antibodies thus resulting in self destruction. The presence of these peculiar antibodies, called 'rheumatoid factor', is detectable in the blood and occurs in most rheumatoid arthritics. The anti-body reaction damages joint membranes which then leads to joint degeneration, and often the improper deposition of calcium. In the later

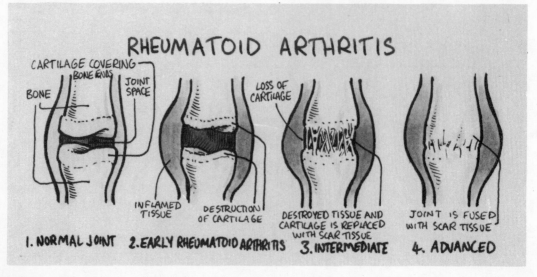

Figure 4.5.3 — *Rheumatoid arthritis*

stages joints may actually fuse together.

While osteoarthritis usually affects the weight-bearing joints, hips, lower back and knees, with variations depending on posture, rheumatoid arthritis usually occurs on both sides of the body and may be localized or general. It often flares up and can be linked to specific allergies, whether connected with food or environment.

The copper connection

The mechanism that leads to destruction of joints involves free ranging oxidizing radicals so it is no surprise to find that the anti-oxidants vitamins A, C, E and selenium often help to relieve symptoms. Manganese, copper and zinc, all involved in the anti-oxidant superoxide dismutases are also important. However, some studies have shown that excessive consumption of iron or copper can cause a flare up of inflammation although not affecting the actual joint degeneration. Since copper is often oversupplied due to its use in water pipes, copper and iron excess should be carefully checked in the rheumatoid arthritic.

Essential fats and arthritis

Prostaglandin series 1, produced from linoleic acid, and prostaglandin series 3, produced from linolenic acid, are both anti-inflammatory. A more direct source of these prostaglandins are gamma-linolenic acid (from evening primrose oil or blackcurrant seed oil) and EPA, in fatty fish. Some arthritics find these substances help reduce inflammation.

Also worth investigating is an extract from the green lipped mussel, a type of mucopolysaccharide. This substance is a natural joint lubricant and constituent of connective tissue. Normally we make enough mucopolysaccharides but with age, these levels drop and are especially low in arthritics. Some early studies have shown that green lipped mussel extract provides relief in 76% of rheumatoid arthritics and 45% of osteo-arthritics. The most effective dose is 1,000mg for the first twenty five days, followed by 250mg a day. It is completely safe and there are no side effects, however some people experience a flare up of symptoms within the first two weeks, before the condition improves. Only people with seafood allergy are advised not to try it.

CHAPTER 4.6

Nutrition, stress and glucose intolerance

—OVERVIEW—

Stress is not an easy word to define, although everybody has a sense of what stress means. Stress means a pressure or tension, created by too many physical, mental or emotional demands. Physiologically our reaction to stress, known as the 'fight or flight syndrome' is a legacy from the days of our ancestors. Situations frequently occurred that required physical action quickly — fight or flight. The body prepares for this rise in effort by diverting blood from the digestive system to the muscles, raising the level of blood sugar, mobilizing fats into the blood stream and increasing pulse and blood pressure. This reaction is caused not only by any type of stress, but by 'adrenal stimulants' such as coffee, alcohol and many other drugs. Refined sugar in the diet has a similar effect in raising blood sugar levels.

Unlike our ancestors, we do not respond with a burst of activity, which is the natural way of utilizing the extra sugar and fats made available, and develop the problem of disposing of the sugar and fats in another way. Insulin is the hormone that is designed for this purpose and is the most important means we have for regulating blood sugar levels. Normally insulin does this well, but if, through repeated adrenal stresses the system is misused, then this regulatory system can malfunction, resulting in one or more forms of glucose intolerance. Diabetes is therefore often a stress-related disease.

The long-term effects of stress and its interaction with nutrition are directly the result of being in 'top gear' too often. This uses up nutrients needed in the stress cycle at an alarming rate. This includes vitamin C, B complex, manganese. zinc and chromium. Stress weakens the immune system increasing the risk of frequent infections, as well as cancer. Stress also interfers with proper digestion, so indigestion and constipation can result.

Stress means pressure or tension — a force exerted in a certain direction. It is the opposite of being at rest or at peace. Excessive stress occurs when the mind, body and emotions are not working together. For example, you have a deadline to meet at work. The mind drives us on and we over-exert the body. The result is stress.

In the body, stress manifests itself as physical tension and the inability to relax. But stress isn't just physical. Emotional upsets, and awkward relationships cause anxiety and mental stress results in preoccupying fears and worries, the mind endlessly chattering without a break. This results in depression.

Every year 46 million prescriptions for anti-depressants, hypnotics and tranquillizers are handed out — drugs designed to block out the fears and worries of modern living. Stress, anxiety and depression is a hidden epidemic.

Whatever its origins, stress has a profound effect on our body chemistry. The heart beats faster and stronger, the blood vessels constrict, the liver converts protein to glucose, muscle cells break down glycogen (stored sugar) to glucose — our whole biochemical orchestra swings into action, conducted by the adrenal glands. But why do we have this potent adrenal system? What, physiologically is the point of the stress reaction?

The evolution of stress

Our ancestors lived in a violent world. They needed to hunt to obtain food, and avoid being hunted. These were their 'stressors', situations that called for bursts of energy. And that, in essence, is what the stress reaction is all about. Providing the muscles with more oxygen and sugar to produce more energy. So refined is our adrenal system that the blood actually coagulates to stop wounds bleeding and natural pain-killers are released, in case of injury. It is the ability to react in stressful situations that helped make man, and other species, dominant. But not only did stress literally save our lives, but we almost became addicted to the stress reaction, liking to fight even when not necessary.

In this context, modern man's behaviour begins to make sense. Why is it we like contact sports, watch murder stories and thrillers on TV, drive around in fast cars, take part in dangerous sports, and get promoted into stressful jobs at the edge of our capacity, while our children play space invaders and watch horror films? The stress reaction can also be turned on by 'adrenal stimulants'. These include sugar, coffee, cigarettes, tea, alcohol and some drugs — again all part of modern living.

Nutritional stressors and their effects on health

ALCOHOL is made by the action of yeast on sugar. As such it has a similar action to glucose metabolism as sugar. Alcohol inhibits the mobilization of reserve glucose from the liver and depresses the demand for more sugar by the hypothalamus, thus contributing to low blood sugar problems. Alcohol interferes with zinc absorption, and encourages the absorption of lead. Excessive consumption greatly increases the risk of diabetes, heart disease, cirrhosis and cancer of the liver.

CHOCOLATE contains cocoa as its major 'active' ingredient. Cocoa provides significant quantities of the stimulant theobromine, whose action is similar although not as strong as caffeine. Cocoa is 1% theobromine, which is also contained in cocoa drinks. A cup of hot chocolate can also contain as much as 5 to 10mg caffeine.

CIGARETTES contain nicotine as well as sixteen cancer-producing chemicals. Nicotine is the primary stimulant and has its effect at small dosages. In large amounts nicotine acts as a sedative. The individual variation in reaction to nicotine is considerable. A recent medical report on addictive drugs lists nicotine as more addictive than heroin.

COFFEE contains theobromine, theophylline and caffeine, all of which act as stimulants. Caffeine is the major stimulant, a cup of coffee containing about 60mg. However, decaffeinated coffee still provides theobromine and theophylline. Theophylline disturbs normal sleep patterns. Coffee consumption is particularly dangerous during pregnancy and breastfeeding as infants are highly susceptible to its effects. Heavy coffee consumption during pregnancy is associated with foetal malformations though there is yet no proof. Children consuming excess caffeine become hyperactive. Withdrawal from caffeine can result in headaches. Heavy coffee consumption may be associated with a greater risk of cancer of the pancreas.

COLA drinks contain between 5 and 7mg of caffeine which is a quarter of that found in a cup of coffee. In addition, these drinks are often high in sugar and colourings and their net stimulant effects can be considerable.

MEDICATIONS provided for the relief of headaches may contain caffeine. Other caffeine tablets are available as stimulants. The most common are Pro Plus and the herb Guarana.

But unlike our ancestors our stresses are mainly mental, emotional and nutritional, not physical. However they cause the same increased availability of sugar and oxygen to the cells eve though we don't need it. Our ancestors would 'burn off'

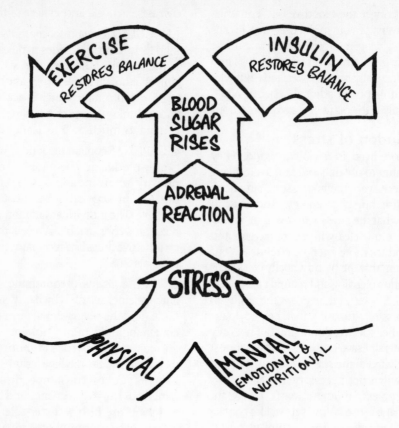

Figure 4.6.1 — *The stress cycle*

this extra fuel, thus restoring balance, but what about us? How do we restore body chemistry to normal?

The stress reaction

Stress has many effects on the body. In the short term it makes all immediate stores of glucose and glycogen available to muscle cells; it stops digestion, and stimulates excretion; stimulates breathing; makes the blood more able to coagulate; releases anti-inflammatory and pain-killer substances; speeds up circulation and raises blood-pressure; and stimulates the pancreas to produce insulin which transports the increased blood sugar levels to the cells.

This all sounds highly desirable but in the long term it's not. Stress causes the body to age by slowing down cell repair; interferes with digestion; slows down metabolism and as the adrenal

glands become exhausted more and more of the stimulant is needed to create the same reaction. So stress, and adrenal stimulants become addictive, like coffee and cigarettes.

Stress and blood sugar

Continuous stress upsets the whole endocrine system (see Chapter 2.3), causing problems of calcium balance, metabolism, sex hormone balance and blood sugar balance. The key organ to be affected is the pancreas. It produces two hormones, insulin and glucagon. Insulin is released whenever blood sugar levels are high and helps transport the sugar to cells. Another substance, called glucose tolerance factor, is released from the liver and aids insulin in its work. If the blood sugar level drops too low the pancreas releases glucagon to stimulate the liver to break down more glycogen to make glucose.

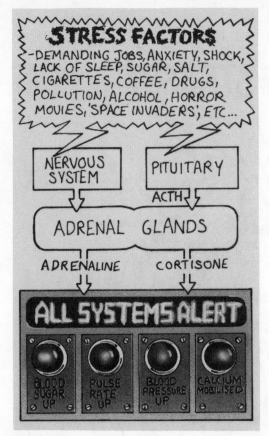

Figure 4.6.2 — *Stress reaction*

palpitations, muscle cramps, excess sweating, digestive problems, allergies, blurred vision, lack of sex drive, thirst.

When blood sugar drops too low this is called hypoglycaemia (hypo = low, glyc = sugar, aemia = in the blood). This can occur as a result of not having eaten, or taken a stimulant recently. This is called functional hypoglycaemia and symptoms are worst first thing in the morning. Another type of hypoglycaemia occurs as a response to ingesting a wide range of substances. This is called reactive hypoglycaemia and is often the mechanism behind the symptoms of food allergies. All stimulants, including sugar, can cause this 'rebound' effect. So does alcohol and cannabis. Symptoms are therefore worse usually within two hours of ingestion.

The worst form of glucose intolerance may follow hypoglycaemia and that is diabetes. Here the body has become unable to transport sugar from blood to the cells and blood sugar level rises. Sugar may appear in the urine as the kidneys' ability to reabsorb sugar becomes saturated. This is caused by a lack of insulin, defective insulin or a lack of glucose tolerance factor. Diabetes can also occur in children, which is thought to be less to do with diet and more to do with a genetic defect in sugar metabolism.

The anti-stress nutrients

The stress reaction and the sugar cycle are all highly dependent on vitamins and minerals. The adrenal glands are rich in B vitamins and vitamin C, and cortisone, an adrenal hormone, needs vitamin B_5 to be produced. Insulin production is dependent on vitamin B_6 and zinc. Glucose tolerance factor depends on vitamin B_3 and chromium. Calcium and magnesium are also needed for nerve and muscle function. All these nutrients get severely depleted in prolonged stress.

How to reduce stress

While a certain amount of stress or stimulation is beneficial, long-term excessive stress is probably one of the primary causes of disease. It is associated with heart disease, cancer, diabetes, premature ageing, and poor resistance to

If the blood sugar stays low (because immediate sources of sugar have been used up) we feel hungry and eat, or take a stimulant. That's why a cigarette or a coffee can actually suppress the appetite. Alcohol, however, doesn't have this effect. In the short term alcohol actually lowers blood sugar and so can stimulate the appetite.

Stress causes glucose intolerance

The use of stimulants or prolonged stress leads to an inability to control blood sugar levels. If the blood sugar level goes too high, drops too low or even rises or falls too rapidly both brain and body become imbalanced as cells are starved or flooded with sugar. The symptoms include irritability, aggressive outbursts, nervousness, depression, crying spells, vertigo and dizziness, fears and anxiety, forgetfulness, inability to concentrate, fatigue, insomnia, headaches,

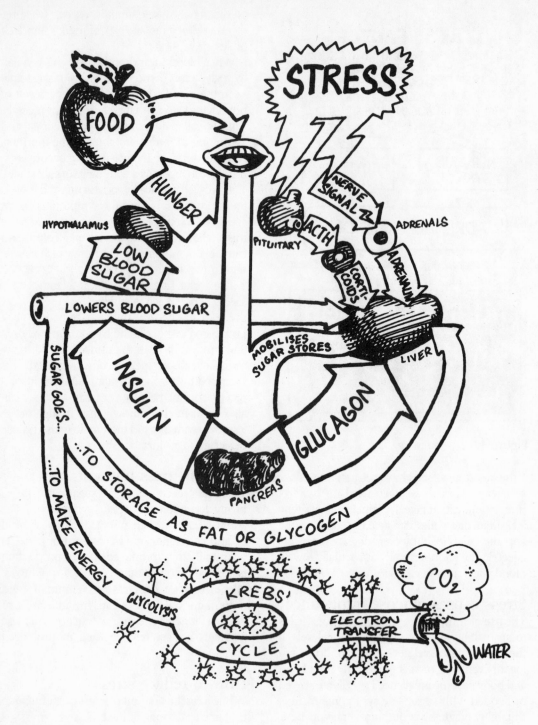

Figure 4.6.3 — *Sugar cycle*

infection. Here are ten tips to make sure your level of stress is not too much.

Limit your working hours to, at most, ten hours a day, five days a week.

Keep at least one and a half days a week completely free of routine work.

Make sure you use this free time to cultivate a relaxing hobby, do something creative or take exercise, preferably in the fresh air.

Try to adopt a relaxed manner. For instance walk and talk more slowly. A useful idea is to act 'as if' you were a relaxed person, almost as a game.

Avoid obvious pressures, such as taking on too many commitments.

Learn to see when a problem is somebody else's responsibility and refuse to take it on.

If you have an emotional problem you cannot solve alone, seek advice.

Concentrate on one task at a time, and focus all your attention on the present.

Learn to say what is on your mind instead of suppressing it. You don't have to be aggressive — just to state your point of view clearly.

Listen to what other people say to you, and about you.

Look long and hard at all the stresses in your life. Make a list of them.

Breathing exercises are also excellent for maintaining a low level of stress.

To maximize your resistance to stress avoid all stimulants, especially when stressed. When you are relaxed, perhaps on holiday, away from the pressures of work, these stimulants will be less harmful. But when stressed they are best avoided completely. Also increase your intake of the anti-stress vitamins.

CHAPTER 4.7

Nutrition and weight control

—OVERVIEW—

More than half the population are classed as overweight. Of these, a proportion are obese, technically defined as more than 20% above their ideal weight. For these people being overweight increases their risk of a number of diseases, among them cardiovascular disease, cancer and diabetes. For a significant proportion of the others, being overweight is a problem of image.

But why do we become overweight, particularly in later years? And why is it so hard to lose weight? The extra undesirable weight is fat, which is our means for storing energy from eating more food than needed. We can express food intake in units of potential energy, called a calorie. A kilocalorie is the amount of energy required to raise one kilogram of water one degree centigrade. The average daily requirement in terms of calories is around 2,500 kcals. When we speak of calories in our diet it is really kilocalories that we are referring to. A certain amount of these calories will be used up by the body simply in maintaining normal body processes. This is called the basal metabolic rate. The rest will be used up through activities: walking, lifting, exercising and so on.

If more food in terms of energy is eaten than is expended the surplus goes to fat. Some people can afford to eat more food because their bodies have a higher basal metabolic rate. Others have a low metabolic rate and get fat even on 2,000 calories diets. So there are three parts to the weight equation. Food in, exercise out and metabolism in the middle.

Most diets concentrate on ways of eating less calories. For example, crash liquid diets, high fibre diets and mono diets all restrict calories. Some diets include foods thought harder to metabolize, such as high protein diets, which are less efficiently converted into energy. Few diets aim to stimulate and balance metabolism.

In addition to problems of obesity, a growing number of mainly young women are developing eating disorders which either compel them to be thinner than is consistent with health — anorexia nervosa — or which involve bingeing followed by voluntary vomiting — anorexia bulimia. All forms of weight problems share a loss of appropriate appetite for maintaining a consistent weight.

Armed with calories charts and even calories calculators countless people have performed mathematical equations over breakfast, lunch and dinner. Although the most popular approach to weight loss, calorie counting is not without its difficulties, nor its failures. Low calories diets are, in practice, hard to stick to and often cause a low metabolic rate, which results in a rebound effect on weight once the diet is over.

The calorie content in food varies according to the type of food. Fat is most calorific (9 kcals per gram), followed by protein (4 kcals) then carbohydrate (3.75 kcals). On the other side of the balance, different activities use up different amounts of calories. For example, an hour of walking uses up 200 calories, while half an hour of energetic cycling may use up 250 calories. If you eat more than you burn off in activity you get fat, and if you eat less than you burn off you get thin. At least that's the theory.

The problems with calories theory

According to Dr Colgan, author of *Your Personal Vitamin Profile*,[47] some of the athletes he works with burn off over 7,000 calories, but eat only 3,500 calories. By calorie theory, these athletes should have disappeared completely by now. An investigation by Dr Apfelbaum of people living in famine in the Warsaw ghetto during the Second World War, shows the same contradiction. With an average calorie intake of 700-800 calories per day, and a daily requirement of say 2.500 calories, a deficit of 1,241,000 calories would build up over two years. The average body has thirty pounds of fat, representing 100,000 calories, to dispose of. Even if all this fat were lost, what happened to the remaining 1 million calories?

Since 1lb of fat is roughly equivalent to 4,000 calories, eating 40,000 calories less per year would mean losing 10lbs in the first year, three and a half stone by the fifth year, over seven stone by the tenth year and vanish entirely after fifteen years! All by eating two less apples every day. Because two apples provide 100 calories a day or 36,500 a year. Turn the equation round the other way, and the simple sin of two extra daily apples would mean a gain of seven stone every ten years.

Even though calories theory doesn't completely add up many people do lose weight and keep it off through low calorie diets.

Very low calories diets

Known as VLCLs there now exist many 'liquid' diets which aim to restrict calorie intake to 330 calories while providing at least RDA levels of all vitamins and minerals. These crash diets are intended to cause a rapid weight loss in one or two weeks. The presence of vitamins and minerals in levels higher than that which most people obtain from diet alone may explain positive reports of well-being on these diets and weight is definitely lost. However, on such a low calorie diet it is likely that both fat and lean muscle tissue is lost also. Since crash dieting also lowers metabolic rate, and since it is lean muscle that consumes more calories than fat, the long-term results of these diets is far less spectacular than the short-term instant weight loss.

The problems with calories theory are not just mathematical ones. Proponents of calorie theory, like Audrey Eyton, author of The F-Plan Diet,[48] have realized that the major problem to calorie controlled diets is that people get hungry. The question became 'How can we eat 1,000 calories a day and feel satisfied?'. The answer was fibre.

The high fibre approach

Fibre is a natural constituent of a healthy diet high in fruits, vegetables, nuts, seeds and grains. Because it absorbs water high fibre diets give the feeling of fullness even though less calories may have been eaten. It is well known that those on high fibre diets have less risk of bowel cancer, diabetes, or diverticular disease, as well as relieving constipation.

Fibre is also relatively calorie free and there is little doubt that a diet high in fibre is more satisfying and easier to follow. After all, which would you find easier to eat: two sweet biscuits, or a pound of carrots?

However, the results of weight loss on diets high in cereal fibre, like bran, are not that spectacular. It is also wiser to eat more raw vegetables (our primary source of fibre), whole grains and fruit, rather than adding bran to a fibre poor diet. Bran contains a high level of phytate, which reduces our absorption of some essential minerals, including zinc. On a wholefood diet these minerals are well supplied. On a junk food diet they are not, and simply adding bran may tip the scales towards deficiency.

While we have learnt that low calorie diets do help maintain correct weight and that high fibre content in the diet makes this easier, there are many more pieces of the jigsaw.

Glucomannan fibre

One of the keys to balancing metabolism is to prevent rapid increases or drops in levels of sugar (which is what all carbohydrate food breaks down to) in the blood-stream. Rapid changes can result in increased appetite and food cravings, and conversion of sugar to fat. That's where glucomannan fibre comes in. Unlike ordinary fibre, glucomannan fibre helps to stabilize blood sugar levels, reducing appetite and balancing metabolic rate. It is also highly absorbent. While bran absorbs ten times its volume in water, glucomannan absorbs 100 times its volume. Only three grams of glucomannan fibre per day have been shown to produce substantial weight loss (at least 6lbs in three months) without any change in exercise or quantity of food eaten.

Eat fat, grow slim?

Advocates of high-fat, low carbohydrate diets believe that if you don't eat carbohydrate you must burn fat instead. Fat is, after all, a very good form of fuel, giving twice as much energy per gram. But burning fat is a bit like lighting a log with a match — it doesn't work. You need kindling to get a good 'fat' fire burning and carbohydrate is the kindling. So just like a fire that smokes because it burns inefficiently, a high fat diet gives off smoke in the form of 'ketones'. High-fat theorists claim that this inefficient metabolism means a loss of potential fat calories as ketones are excreted. But other scientists beg to differ. Research has clearly established that, at most, 100 to 150 kcals are lost in ketone excretion and what is more worrying excessive ketone levels are extremely dangerous.[49]

High protein diets

High protein, low carbohydrate diets are also to be avoided for health reasons. By restricting carbohydrate intake, inefficient fat breakdown may occur, again causing an increase in ketones. Protein may also be used for fuel, and the advocate of this approach argues that protein is hard to convert and therefore less calories are consumed by the body at the end of the day. There may be an element of truth in this, but any diet which aims to imbalance metabolism is at best a short-term answer and at worst positively bad for your health. After all, fifty-eight deaths in the USA have been associated with low calorie, high protein diets.

Fasting diets

Modified fasts are the most severe approach to dieting. For those with life-threatening obesity they may be of value, but they are certainly not for the average person. One study followed 207 patients hospitalized for fasting over nine years. While seventy nine reduced their weight to within 30% of their ideal weight, 90% of these were back to their original weight nine years later. Hardly a long-term solution.

Starch blockers don't work

'Just swallow these pills and they'll stop you digesting starch, so you can eat as much as you like without getting fat.' That was the argument put forward in 1983 when sales of starch blocker tablets rocketed throughout the world. Dr Hollenbeck studied the effects of these starch blockers and found no evidence of any effect on carbohydrate metabolism.[50] He also found very variable levels of the starch enzyme inhibitor, as well as lectin which is a potentially dangerous substance in beans, from which the raw material was derived. Lectin is destroyed in cooking. The only significant physiological changes these pills had was an increase in flatulence!

Raising metabolic rate

Probably the most important key to understanding weight gain and promoting weight loss is the changes that occur in metabolic rate. By increasing metabolic rate and changing diet so you're eating more in quantity but a little less in calories the net effect has to be weight loss. To understand how to increase your metabolism let us consider how metabolism works.

Everything you eat (except vitamins and minerals) can be divided into fat, protein or carbohydrate. All of these can be converted by the body into fat or energy. This transition happens through a series of chemical reactions, activated by enzymes, which are dependent upon different vitamins and minerals. But not all types of food are easy to convert into energy. Some require more energy to initiate the chemical reactions than others.

Quality *vs* quantity in diets

Ideally, we eat protein for one reason only — that is to replace old body cells. We don't need it for energy. Carbohydrates are our most ideal fuel. Too much protein is hard work for the body to eliminate. But if fat provides more calories, surely it's a better energy source than carbohydrate? If our bodies were simply energy machines this would be true, but they're not and too much fat has its problems. First of all, since fat is higher in calories its easier to eat more of it and put on weight. What's more, the higher the level of fat circulating in your bloodstream, the greater the risk of heart disease, diabetes and kidney disease to start with. Too much fat means the body has to break it down and get rid of the excess. There are a number of stages that can go wrong, and the result may be extra work for the kidneys or a build up of fats in the blood and in the artery walls.

But fat is not all bad. We've got to get some essential fatty acids, otherwise we get ill. These EFAs are found mainly in the leaves and seeds of plants, and are also high in fish. We also need some fat to help absorb the fat soluble vitamins. The fat on our bodies, which acts as padding, can be made from dietary fat or carbohydrates.

Carbohydrates are the best kind of energy food. A carbohydrate, for example potato, is broken down through a series of chemical reactions, the end product being glucose, which is the simplest carbohydrate called a sugar. This takes place over a matter of hours and provides us with a gradual supply of energy. You might think then why not just eat glucose, or other simple sugars like sucrose (white table sugar), or fructose (fruit sugar)? It is the gradual release of glucose into the blood-stream, controlled by enzymes acting on complex carbohydrates, that helps provide us with a constant supply of fuel for energy. Coupled with a good supply of vitamins and minerals metabolic rate remains high. However too much simple sugar and blood sugar level becomes imbalanced. So does metabolism. So a high complex carbohydrate diet is consistent with a good metabolic rate.

Vitamins and minerals and metabolism

However, diet alone is not enough. Many vitamins, and also minerals are needed for proper metabolism. Anecdotal evidence suggests that, taken as supplements, a combination of vital nutrients helps to boost metabolic rate and assist weight loss. Twenty-two vitamins and minerals are needed for proper metabolism and weight control. Although our needs vary from person to person, ten of these are vital for improving metabolism and helping to break down fat. These are vitamin B_1, B_2, B_3, pantothenic acid, B_6, C, choline, inositol, chromium and zinc.

This is what the most important ones do

B_6 is fundamental for the production of pancreatic enzymes, which ensure smooth digestion. It is also needed for the production and regulation of sex hormones and adrenalin and helps produce brain chemicals involved with our moods. B_6 is best taken with zinc. 100mg to 300mg per day are recommended.

B_3 (nicotinic acid) is one of the constituents of GTF (see chromium) needed to maintain our blood sugar balance. It is essential for converting unused glucose to glycogen, the body's short-term reservoir of energy. In doses of 1gm B_3 lowers cholesterol levels. Normally 50 to 250mg per day are quite adequate.

Vitamin C has many roles to play in weight control. Firstly, it is needed for hormone production in the adrenal glands and is a vital link to preventing glandular exhaustion leading to slow metabolism. It is involved in the conversion of glucose to energy in the cell. Like B_3 it also lowers elevated cholesterol levels. The recommended daily dose is 1 to 3g.

Chromium is the major nutrient in GTF (Glucose Tolerance Factor) released every time our blood sugar level rises. GTF makes insulin more effective and is therefore crucial for balanced blood sugar levels. Chromium is widely deficient, especially among the elderly. 20 to 100mcg are recommended daily.

Zinc is probably the most deficient mineral in Britian. It is involved in over twenty different enzyme reactions, including the energy cycle. Zinc deficiency disturbs sense of taste and smell, as well as appetite. Deficiency of zinc is also associated with stretch marks, poor wound healing, poor eyesight and may be involved in anorexia nervosa and bulimia. In case you're wondering, becoming zinc deficient is not the way to lose weight! 15 to 25mg are needed each day. But the average diet provides only 9 to 11mg and even less if you're a vegetarian.

Exercise and metabolic rate

The good news about exercise is that you really don't have to be fanatically fit to lose weight. And the reason why is not calories, it's metabolism. According to the calorie theory, exercise doesn't do much to promote weight loss. After all, a three mile run only burns up 300 calories. That's equivalent to two slices of toast or a piece of apple pie. But this argument, upon which has hinged the preference to eat less rather than exercise more to lose weight, misses four important facts.

The first is that the effects of exercise are cumulative. Running a mile may only burn up 300 calories, but if you do that three days a week for a year that's 22,000 calories, equivalent to a weight loss of 11 pounds! Also, the amount of calories you burn up depends upon how fat you are to start with, how hard and how long you exercise and how much of you is fat or muscle. For example, consider someone who weighs 14 stone compared to someone weighing 9 stone. If the 14 stone person runs one mile in 8 minutes, and the 9 stone person does it in 10 minutes, the heavier person will use up over 1,000 calories, and the lighter person will only burn up 500 calories.

However, a fat person won't lose much weight to start with from exercise. Because first of all that fatty muscle tissue gets converted to lean muscle tissue. With extra muscle you can burn off that excess fat faster and faster. So even though you may not lose weight with exercise to begin

with you are replacing fat with muscle and becoming less fat, and that's what counts for long-term weight loss.

Another myth about exercise is that you can keep fit through housework. In fact, a sedentary worker or houseperson will burn up around 2,000 calories a day. Reducing intake to 1,750 calories a day would not have a substantial effect. However, even small but regular amounts of exercise make all the difference.

For example, one study examined the effects of walking on six overfat and underfit young men. Five days a week for sixteen weeks they walked for 90 minutes a day. That's the equivalent of 45 minutes to work and back. They lost an average of 12.5lbs, their percentage of body fat dropped from 23.5% to 18.6% and their blood fat levels improved, which is a measure of heart health. That means that if you could walk the last fifteen minutes to work and back you would lose 14lbs in a year, without making any extra effort to exercise.

Exercise decreases appetite

Contrary to popular belief, moderate exercise actually decreases your appetite. Both animals and man consistently show decreased appetite with small increases in physical activity. One study looked at an industrial population in West Bengal, India. Those doing sedentary work ate more and consequently weighed more than those doing light work. As the level of work increased from light to heavy workers ate more, but not relative to their energy output. The result was that the heavier the work the lighter the worker.

Effect of exercise on calorie intake and body weight

Job Classification	Daily Calorie Intake (kcal)	Body Weight (lbs)
Sedentary	3,300	148
Light work	2,600	118
Medium work	2,800	114
Heavy work	3,400	113
Very heavy work	3,600	113

It appears that a degree of physical activity is necessary for appetite mechanisms to work properly. Those who do not exercise have exaggerated appetites and hence the pounds gradually creep on.

Exercise boosts metabolic rate

But the most important reason why exercise is a key to weight loss is its effect on your metabolic rate. According to Professor McArdle, exercise physiologist at City University,[49] New York

> Most people can generate metabolic rates that are eight to ten times above the resting value during sustained running, cycling or swimming. Complementing this increased metabolic rate is the observation that vigorous exercise will raise the metabolic rate for up to fifteen hours after exercise.

In fact, other studies have shown that metabolic rate is raised by 25% for fifteen hours and by 10% for forty-eight hours. According to sports physiologist Professor Fenton

> Exercise has a stimulating effect on metabolism which persists throughout the day, raising metabolic rate and leading to the loss of appreciably more fat than would have been predicted for the exercise taken.

The metabolic effect of the exercise is far more significant than the calories used up in the exercise itself. Simply by doing 12 minutes of aerobic exercise a day you can substantially increase your metabolic rate, without increasing your appetite. The net result is weight loss.

Anorexia and nutrition

Despite claims to the contrary there is little doubt that in most cases of anorexia nervosa (chronic undereating resulting in loss of weight) and anorexia bulimia (bingeing followed by voluntary vomiting) psychological factors play a significant part. Anorexia often occurs as a result of grief or as a resistance in young girls to becoming adults. By restricting eating, periods stop and other sexual characteristics also diminish. However there are many other potential causes for these problems.

With restricted eating protein, vitamin and mineral deficiency is prevalent. The lack of these essential nutrients impairs nerve and brain function, further promoting emotional instability.

Deficiency of B vitamins and of zinc is also consistent with disturbance in appetite. So there comes a point where the mind and body are both imbalanced and a vicious cycle develops. Without meaning to explore the complex nature of these conditions a nutritionist must first seek to restore nutritional balance. This is first best achieved by restoring vitamin and mineral levels through diet and supplements, particularly ensuring adequate zinc status. Since supplements are not considered as food, and hence won't induce weight gain, these are often best accepted by the anorexic, aware there is a problem, feeling low in energy and suffering from poor circulation, but still not wishing to put on weight.

As nutritional status improves this often induces more physical and mental well-being thereby supporting the individual in coming to terms with any underlying problems. In some documented cases of anorexia the supplementation of zinc alone has produced a complete recovery, so the conclusion of a psychogenic origin to this problem should not be assumed without investigation of nutritional deficiencies.

Binge eating

Patterns of binge eating are often indicative of either blood sugar imbalances or food allergies. Many people have the experience of only bingeing on certain foods. For example, although they like apples and biscuits, on eating one biscuit the whole packet is eaten. The same craving does not usually exist for apples.

If you are allergic to a particular food, you are likely to crave that food and therefore eat it frequently. It's as if you are mildly addicted. Through working with a number of allergic and overweight clients, it became clear that bingeing, or uncontrolled overeating, often happened only with certain food groups. When clients were instructed to eat as much as they like of anything but not the suspected allergen (food that provokes an allergic reaction), bingeing often ceased completely. When the allergen was totally avoided clients sometimes lost as much as 7lbs weight overnight. This sort of short-term weight loss had to be the result of excess fluid retention and nothing to do with fat.

One of the physical symptoms of an allergic reaction can be sudden fluctuations in blood sugar level. This in turn affects appetite. Could it be that the initial allergic reaction to the food was setting the scene for increased appetite and hence bingeing? In honesty, nobody has a definite answer to this question, but my observations with a number of clients certainly show that sometimes allergies do play a role in overweight problems.

PART FIVE

——— INDIVIDUAL NUTRITION ———

CHAPTER 5.1

Nutrition for the elderly

—OVERVIEW—

If it is important to pay attention to nutritional factors when young, then it is doubly important to get these factors right as we age. Less calories are needed due to a decline in general level of activity, together with a drop in overall metabolic rate. Appetite also declines but for most people this isn't sufficient to reduce the amount of food they eat to a level that will keep their weight constant. Thus obesity is the usual result, together with the increased risk of degenerative disease that it brings.

However just because the need for calories declines with age this does not mean that the need for vitamins and minerals follows the same pattern. Indeed the opposite is usually the case. For some minerals poorly supplied over the years, like chromium, manganese and selenium, levels may be reduced to virtually nothing. For others, like calcium, the mechanism for absorption may have become impaired. Others still, like zinc, are needed to ensure maximum function in the immune system which declines with age. It is this decline in immune power that mkes cells particularly susceptible to free radical damage. Free radicals are potentially mutagenic chemicals that start a chain reaction of destruction, and so an anti-ageing programme includes high levels of the anti-oxidant nutrients, particularly vitamins E, C, and A and the mineral selenium. The brown marks (lipofuscin) in the skin of elderly people are a sign of free radical damage to the skin cells.

On the other hand, anti-nutrients that can store may reach significant levels of concentration in old age. Aluminium, for example, has been found in large quantities in the brains of those with senile dementia. It is strongly implicated in decline in memory in later years.

So as we age there are a whole host of parameters which decline in function, such as stamina, memory, skin condition, immune strength and digestive efficiency. These are the markers of ageing. The rate at which these parameters decline can vary from person to person and are strongly influenced by lifestyle and nutritional factors.

As Leonard Larson, president of the American Medical Association said in 1960, 'There are no diseases of the aged, but simply diseases among the aged'. Likewise, what constitutes the elderly depends more upon the level of health than the chronological age of the individual. In Britain, the average lifespan is seventy-two for men and seventy-six for women. However, the oldest recorded person died at the age of 120, with deteriorating health from 113. However this chapter considers the nutritional needs and diseases of the 'average' elderly person.

Changes in nutritional requirements must be based on age-related changes in the ability of the lungs to take in oxygen, on the effects of atherosclerosis, on reduced absorption of nutrients, and on reduced sense of taste altering self-selection of foods. Also, according to one survey, 59% of women over the age of fifty-nine are more than 20% above their ideal weight, so possible obesity needs also be considered. Also considerable are the reduced efficiency of the immune system, and impaired memory and intellectual capabilities. These factors suggest that the elderly's need for nutrients would be greater than that of a younger person. Due to a reduced metabolic rate and decreased calories output through exercise the elderly tend to require far fewer calories. So that means they need less food and more nutrients.

Vitamin and mineral deficiency is common

It is therefore not so surprising to see that the elderly are the worst nourished section of the population. As an illustration to this point rather than proof, one survey investigated nutritional status in ninety-three unselected admissions to a geriatric hospital. On examining vitamin and mineral levels in the blood only fifteen people had normal blood levels of nutrients. Most common were deficiencies of folic acid, iron, zinc, B_1, B_2 and B_3. Also common, although not well determined from blood, was calcium deficiency. The drop in oestrogen levels after the menopause worsens calcium absorption and makes women particularly susceptible to osteoporosis. Other studies have added vitamin A, C, E, B_6 and B_{12} to this long list.

These deficiences occur not only as a result of faulty diet but also because of poor absorption. For example, in another survey 14% of elderly people found to be anaemic had sufficient diets, according to Recommended Daily Allowances. Calcium, zinc, iron and B_{12} absorption are particularly impaired.

Unfortunately, the decline in zinc status is one factor that accelerates lack of sense of taste and smell. This, in turn, leads to dietary changes away from blander foods such as vegetables, high in nutrients, towards strong tasting foods such as cheese, meat and salted foods. It is therefore not surprising to find that diets tend to be too high in fat. However lowering fat intake may also

further lower zinc and iron.

Many essential trace elements whose status is borderline in the general population become deficient in the elderly simply because the passage of time reduces body stores and at the same time the body absorbs less. Among these are manganese, selenium and chromium. Chromium stores in the body are usually completely depleted by the age of sixty.

Supplementation is essential

To maintain ideal nutrient intake in the elderly, supplementation with vitamins and minerals is essential. The chart below compares normal RDAs for an elderly man (assuming a sedentary life) with the optimum levels and recommended levels for supplementation.

Nutrient	RDA*	Optimum level	Supplemental level
A	2,500iu	10,000iu	7,500iu
D	—	500iu	400iu
E	—	500iu	100iu
C	30mg	3,000mg	3,000mg
B_1	0.9mg	100mg	75mg
B_2	1.6mg	100mg	75mg
B_3	18mg	200mg	200mg
B_5	—	200mg	200mg
B_6	—	100mg	100mg
B_{12}	2mcg	10mcg	10mcg
Folic acid	300mcg	300mcg	100mcg
Choline	—	250mg	250mg
Calcium	500mg	750mg	500mg
Magnesium	—	400mg	300mg
Zinc	—	20mg	15mg
Iron	10mg	15mg	10mg
Chromium	—	50mcg	50mcg
Manganese	—	5mg	5mg
Selenium	—	50mcg	50mcg

Chart 5.1.1 — *Nutritional needs in the elderly*

Toxic elements tend to store and thus accumulate with age. Examples of this are rising lead and aluminium levels with age. While the exposure to these toxic elements may only have been slight the gradual accumulation of these toxic elements poses a real problem for many elderly people. Aluminium for example has been strongly linked to Alzheimer's disease, a type of senility.

Ageing without senility

Senility is described as a 'mental disease in which brain cells cease to function properly, resulting in a deficit in memory and mental capability'.[51] The size of the problem is on the increase. One in four people over seventy-five are classified as senile and one in seven over sixty-five. In fact one third of all hospital beds are filled with geriatrics, a large proportion of them institutionalized because of senility. The cost to the tax payer runs into billions.

To understand senility we must examine the nature of the memory. In a lifetime more than fifteen trillion memories are coded in our brain. Although much of what we perceive is forgotten, selected glimpses remain permanently etched, waiting for recall.

So memory can be divided into short term (lasting a few seconds or minutes) or long term. Computer scientists estimate that to hold all the information in our cabbage-sized brains, it would require a modern computer the size of Buckingham Palace. How do we hold this information? And what goes wrong?

Two current theories exist. One involves coding through lipoproteins, fat-containing proteins in the brain. In fact, every cell in our brain contains special kinds of fat, which can be synthesized only from the essential fatty acids linoleic and linolenic acid. Synthesis of these is made even easier by the intake of fatty fish, high in EPA, or evening primrose oil, high in gamma-linolenic acid.

The other theory is based on coding through RNA, the messenger molecule in charge of building new cells. Since most brain cells are replaced within twenty-four hours, the clue to memory must be transmittable. Foods high in RNA, like fish, have been shown to boost mental activity and memory in animals.

Research at the Brain Bio Center in New Jersey has revealed a link between senile dementia and the protein spermine. Patients with recent memory loss were found to have low levels of spermine — which the brain badly needs to produce more RNA. The minerals zinc and, most importantly, manganese help to bring spermine levels back to normal.[52]

What exactly goes wrong with those suffering from senile dementia? One common finding is that premature senile dementia, known as Alzheimer's disease, is an entanglement of nerve fibres. When these nerve fibres are found in clusters in the frontal and temporal regions of the brain they are frequently loaded with aluminium. It is highly likely that our involuntary consumption of aluminium contributes to deteriorating memory and mental performance. We get aluminium from cooking utensils and food packaging, including aluminium foil. People with indigestion risk an extra dose, from many types of antacids.

Another hypothesis is that nerve cells are simply not getting enough blood supply. Most people, by the age of fifty, have a degree of atherosclerosis — hardening and 'furring up' of the arteries. In severe cases this leads to a stroke, where the whole blood supply to a portion of the brain is cut off. The result is death or partial paralysis.

When cells are starved of oxygen they switch to a more primitive mode of operation called anaerobic respiration. The cells begin to divide and spread. That is, unless they're nerve cells. Because nerve cells can't regenerate. So what happens to them? They just stop working. The result is senility.

Improving oxygen supply

To keep cells running on oxygen requires more than just a good blood supply. Vitamins are also involved in the process of oxygen and energy metabolism. The most important vitamins are B_1 and B_3 and the anti-oxidant nutrients C, E and selenium.

B_1 deficiency has long been known to result in brain damage. One of the most dangerous problems of excessive alcohol consumption is induced B_1 deficiency. The condition is called Wernicke-Korsakoff syndrome. The symptoms include anxiety and depression, obsessive thinking, confusion, defective memory (especially for recent events) and time distortion — not so different from senility.

Vitamin B_3, also known as nicotinic acid or nicotinamide, is crucial for oxygen utilization. It is incorporated into the coenzyme NAD (nicotinamide adenosine dinucleotide), and many reactions involving oxygen need NAD. Without it, pellagra and senility may develop.

CHAPTER 5.2

Nutrition for babies and children

—OVERVIEW—

Babies and children are more susceptible to the effects of sub-optimum nutrition than adults because they are still growing. Also, the younger the child the more immature are its mechanisms for avoiding infections and pollutants and the more susceptible they are to developing allergies, which may go away in time.

Food allergies can result in an enormous variety of different symptoms. In children, behavioural problems, asthma and general ill-health are most common. Hyperactivity can be directly caused by a particular food or food component. Food additives have been implicated here and a special additive free diet (known as the Feingold diet) has been shown to help parents with the problem. Allergies don't develop in children as a matter of chance, and there are several ways in which parents can help them from occurring. Breast milk contains an essential antibody (known as IgA) which helps prevent the baby's immune system from reacting to foods. Thus breast feeding for at least six months is a good preventive step. Similarly a nutritious whole food diet will help the child develop a strong immune system.

Lead and other toxic metals can have an extremely detrimental effect on child development. As well as being a cause of hyperactivity and general ill-health, lead can also retard intelligence. This occurs because lead passes more easily in the brain of young children and does more damage as the brain is still forming. The vast majority of lead contamination comes from car exhausts either directly through breathing or indirectly through eating foods contaminated with lead. Young children are forever putting dirty objects in their mouths which is a considerable source of lead.

Because of their requirements for rapid growth children need proportionately more calcium, magnesium, vitamin D and zinc.

Breast is best

Seventy years ago this chapter would not have been needed, as breastfeeding was the norm. However the number of women who choose to breastfeed has declined so much that now women have to be persuaded back into it. There are many advantages to breast feeding, the most important one being nutritional. Although we have advanced slightly from the days when cow's milk was boiled, diluted and had sugar added to it, we have still not produced a formula milk that is identical to human milk.

Formulas do not contain selenium, important for the prevention of heart disease and cancer, or chromium, needed to produce the glucose tolerance factor. The manganese in breast milk is twenty times more absorbable than that in formula milk. Formulas for tiny babies are sweetened with lactose, as is breast milk, however once a baby is over four months old the sweetener used is corn syrup. This will provide glucose which is a much more readily absorbed form of sugar.

Different milks from different mammals vary enormously. For instance whale milk is so high in fat (and calories) that it resembles double cream. This enables the baby whale to develop a thick layer of blubber to protect it from the cold sea. The initial reasons for giving babies cow's milk half a century ago are very dubious, as, in fact donkey's milk resembles human milk far more closely. Cows were, however, much more available and produce more milk.

Once feeding is established it is far more convenient than messing around with bottles. The baby is far less likely to get gastroenteritis and the risk of developing an allergy to cow's milk is reduced as the baby's gut will leak whole cow's milk molecules. However, the nutritional value of breastfeeding depends very much on the health and nutritional status of the mother.

The pros and cons of breast feeding

There are many more advantages than disadvantages to breastfeeding. For example, during the first vital weeks of life your baby's main protection against disease is obtained from the antibodies found in breast milk — these are not put in formula milk. There is even some evidence that the incidence of cot deaths is higher among bottle-fed babies, particularly during the time of change between breast and bottle. However it is not known why. Breast milk is easier to digest — this could be a contributing factor.

Sucking on a breast is also much harder work than sucking on a bottle, therefore breastfed babies develop a much stronger jaw, which stands them in good stead for later on when you are giving them salad to chew on!

Why breastfeeding helps you to lose weight

On the right diet many women find they lose weight while breastfeeding without any risk of poor nourishment for themselves or their babies. While the US RDA for a lactating woman is 2750 kcals, in one study forty-five lactating women on a 2,186 calories diet remained perfectly healthy, full of energy and produced sufficient breast milk. Their weight after four months dropped by a little over 11 pounds. Their babies grew just as fast as other mothers whose calories intake was higher. Provided the quality of food is good, losing weight during lactation is compatible with successful breastfeeding.

Breastfeeding doesn't guarantee good nutrition

However, mother's milk is only as good as the mother, and most mothers' nutrition is far from good enough to guarantee the baby the best start in life. For instance, take vitamin B_6 levels in milk. An infant needs 0.3mg per day according to the US recommended daily allowance. A group of women whose diets were analysed to contain on average 1.8mg a day, which is marginally below the RDA of 2mg, were given varying levels of B_6 supplementation, from nothing up to 20mg, which is ten times higher than the RDA. The levels of B_6 found in breast milk provided the equivalent of 0.06mg for those unsupplemented, up to 0.28mg for those supplementing an extra 20mg a day. In other words, even this level of supplementation didn't meet the baby's basic needs for B_6. Supplements of 50mg of B_6 are recommended in pregnancy to reach optimal levels. However a word of caution. Doses in excess of 200 to 600mg per day have been reported to suppress lactation. There is no danger of this at the 50mg level. However not all B vitamins need to be supplemented in such relatively large amounts. Provided folic acid is supplemented during pregnancy it appears likely that breastfed babies will be getting enough. In a study in which pregnant women supplemented 1,000mcg of folic acid, some continuing for the first three months of lactation, others not, all breast milk analyses indicated that the baby was getting enough.

Babies don't become 'vitamin dependent'

Although some people mistakenly feel that mothers taking large amounts of vitamin C might somehow pass on a vitamin C dependency to the newborn baby, unlike vitamin B_6, there appears to be a mechanism that stops the baby getting more than it needs. The breast milk of mothers supplementing 1,000mg or more of vitamin C provides between 40mg and 86mg daily for the infant. Taking more vitamin C didn't increase the level in breast milk although the mother's excretion of vitamin C did increase.[54] So at least as far as the baby is concerned 1,000mg of vitamin C a day is adequate for the mother.

Breast milk is better for fat soluble vitamins

Vitamin E is one vitamin that comes out on top in breast milk.

Another study has shown that breast milk is higher in vitamin D than ordinary milk. The researchers also identified a particular kind of vitamin D called 25-OHD, which has been shown to be two and a half times more effective for preventing rickets, indicating its more potent effect on increasing calcium utilization. Vitamin D helps to increase calcium supply in the baby by encouraging the absorption of calcium from the gut. This special form of vitamin D is naturally present in breast milk. The suggestion from this research is that this more active form of vitamin D should be added to infant formulas.

Breast milk is zinc deficient

A newborn infant up to six months needs 3mg of zinc a day. Yet the average amount supplied daily in human milk is only 1.3mg during the first three months and even less, only 0.6mg a day in the last three months of breastfeeding. This indicates just how hard it is to provide adequate zinc for the baby. Mothers and babies alike become increasingly deficient as breastfeeding continues. This conclusion has been confirmed in a study that investigated the effects on zinc status of sixteen nursing mothers and the weight and zinc excretion of their exclusively breastfed babies. Those with lower birth weight babies had low serum levels of zinc and the babies tended to excrete less zinc, presumably indicating a greater need.[55]

However, breast milk zinc is generally far better absorbed than dietary zinc, so these low figures may not be as bad as they seem. It may well be the breast feeding mother who suffers more from slight zinc deficiency than the baby. The biggest danger to zinc supply to the baby is prolonged breastfeeding when the mother is on an inadequate diet. Research has clearly shown that breast milk concentrations drop substantially throughout breastfeeding to well below 50% of the RDA for infants. There is little doubt that a breastfeeding mother needs to get at least 25mg of zinc a day, and that means supplementing at least 15mg.

Selenium and breast milk

Selenium is another mineral that is needed in greater amount during pregnancy. Some countries like Finland have poor soil levels of selenium and poor dietary intakes. Studies on Finnish women have shown clearly that on a diet containing 30mcg of selenium a day, breast milk levels of selenium decline as breast feeding continues, and that higher dietary intake increases breast milk levels.[56] Studies of selenium levels in placenta and amniotic tissue show levels three times higher than those in the mother's blood. The suggestion here is that selenium deficiency for the baby is avoided at all costs during pregnancy, including depriving the mother of this essential nutrient. The intake of selenium in Britain is around 60mcg, although a significant number of people get less than 30mcg a day. The suggested daily intake for selenium, which has no RDA in Britain, is 50 to 200mcg. A daily supplement of 50mcg is therefore recommended during lactation.

Which formulas are best?

Not all women have the choice whether or not to breast feed their babies. So which formula is best? Rather than list the many different makes it's better to know what to look for. Firstly you'll want to avoid formulas that contain added sugar, glucose. It simply isn't needed. Then it's a matter of comparing nutrient content. Probably the easiest way to pick out a good formula milk is to compare the zinc content. It should also contain manganese, chromium and selenium, although many don't. The protein content should be broken down into individual amino acids. In America the amino acid taurine, now thought to be essential for babies, is often added. This is another hallmark of a better formula.

Is goat's milk better than cow's milk?

Goat's milk is thought to be less allergenic than cows milk, and some people recommend it instead of cow's milk for baby food. But goat's milk is not ideal on a number of counts. Firstly, most goat's milk is unpasteurized and the risk of infection on a child up to one year is simply not worth it. Secondly, like cow's milk the concentrations of folic acid, vitamin C and D are too low. From the nutrition point of view it is little different from cow's milk. However, some goat's milk is less contaminated with drugs, and if boiled or pasteurized and obtained from animals tested for brucellosis or tuberculosis it is perfectly safe, provided it is diluted and fortified with lactose and folic acid.

Another alternative used in formula milks for children with milk allergy is soya milk. Soya has often been criticized for its poor absorbable zinc. This was thought to be due to the presence of phytate which inhibits zinc uptake. However it may be the high iron content, not the phytate that competes with zinc. Studies have shown than when twice as much iron as zinc is eaten, this inhibits zinc. Soy-formulas contain much more iron than zinc, because even more is added to these formulas. Infants consuming iron enriched soy-formulas do have lower zinc levels. The ideal zinc/iron ratio in breast milk and presumably in diet is around 1:1. Given that some pregnant women ar given 60mg of iron, and only get 9mg of zinc from their diet, there's a long way to go before baby milk formulas could be considered well balanced all round.

Weaning — when and what?

Nature provides babies with their first teeth at around six months and this seems the most sensible (approximate) age to start weaning. The chewing on a crust of wholemeal bread, piece of cucumber or raw carrot will help the other teeth to come through. Another pointer for when to wean is if the baby starts feeding every two hours and this goes on for more than five days. This can indicate that he is not getting the amount of milk he needs and for some reason your supply isn't responding to the demand. Also if a baby who had been sleeping through the night, suddenly starts waking in the night for a feed, this could be the time to introduce a small amount of solid food for his or her dinner.

No baby should be given any solids before four months old, as there is a high possibility that allergies will be induced due to the lack of maturity of the digestive tract. Also most of the food will be going in one end and out of the other, again due to lack of maturity. However, all babies should be on some solids by eight months as the risk of infection has been shown to be higher in babies fed exclusively on breast milk past this age. The baby's iron stores will also be getting low by this age, as there is some iron in breast milk but not enough to provide all the baby's needs. A premature baby may run out of iron stores earlier than a full term baby, so monitoring iron levels in a premature baby is sensible.

The baby's first food

Healthy babies, as with healthy adults, should be fed on food that is fresh, unprocessed, additive-free, sugar-free, (and that includes glucose, dextrose, sucrose, maltose and fructose) and salt-free. In other words food that is close to how it is found in nature. The baby will eventually be eating the food that you eat, so he or she will need to get used to eating this way right from the start. Packaged baby foods are improving all the time, they do not now contain artificial additives and some are sugar free (Heinz do some pure fruit purées that are just that and useful as a stand-by). As with adult food, if you are going to use the odd prepared food, read the label — if it contains any cereal it should be wholemeal and unrefined, it should not contain any of the sugars listed above, modified starch or hydrolized vegetable protein or any ingredient that you do not understand.

Fibre for babies

Some mothers will not give their baby a high fibre diet as it 'goes straight through them'. What they often mean is they are getting three dirty nappies a day and cannot be bothered changing them all that often. As with an adult a healthy bowel should be emptying itself two or three times a day and much of the food will come out as recognizable lentils or grape skins. Much of this is due to the fact that a baby cannot chew foods properly

Preventing allergies

At the start of weaning babies need food that is very easily digested and that is unlikely to cause an allergic reaction. Cooked, puréed vegetables and fruits are a good start. If a fruit or vegetable can be given raw then leave it raw, for example bananas, avocados, very ripe William's pears or paw paws. The later a food is introduced the less likelihood there is of producing an allergic reaction. so if you suspect your child may react allergically (a family history of allergy) or you just want to be absolutely certain that your child does not have any allergies, introduce potential allergens as late as you can. Below is a list of foods and food groups with those most likely to give an allergic reaction at the bottom. So start by giving the foods at the top and as each one is cleared move down the list.

Vegetables except tomatoes, potatoes, aubergines and peppers
Fruits except oranges
Nuts and seeds
Pulses and beans
Rice
Meat
Oats, barley and rye
*Vegetables excluded above
*Oranges
*Wheat
*Milk products
*Eggs

Chart 5.2.1 — *Low allergenic foods (in descending order)*

Introduce one or two foods each day and make a note of which foods you have given and any possible reaction. A reaction may be anything from severe to mild eczema, excessive sleepiness, a runny nose, an ear infection, excessive thirst, over-activity or asthmatic breathing. If you notice a reaction withdraw that food and carry on with new foods once the reaction has died down. You can double check your observations a few months later, the reaction may also disappear as the digestive system matures. The five starred foods should not be introduced until nine or ten months — this also applies to any foods that either the mother or father is known to react to.

A newly weaned baby will still be getting a large amount of nourishment from breast milk and the mother may well be breastfeeding as much as before. This is quite all right, in fact it is to be encouraged. Assuming the baby is getting most of his protein, fat and carbohydrate from milk, it would be best to feed a baby plenty of vitamin and mineral rich vegetables and fruit. These are very easy to prepare — just cook a combination of vegetables or fruit, no need to add sugar, and purée in a liquidizer, food processor, mouli or special baby food blender. Here are some suggestions for good combinations:

BABY FOOD PURÉES
Carrots — alone

Cauliflower and turnip

Carrots, spinach and cauliflower

Broad beans and cauliflower or carrot and a very little celery

Jerusalem artichokes and carrot

Peeled courgettes (the skins can be bitter) and fennel

Leek and potato

Swede, turnip and potato

As time goes on other ingredients like red split lentils, cooked bean sprouts, well-cooked brown rice, black-eyed beans and other pulses, milk, cheese, yogurt or soya milk.

Breakfasts can be more puréed vegetables. They do not have to be sweet cereals or fruit. This is an unnecessary way to educate a sweet tooth from a very early age. As cereals are introduced into the diet, you can cook brown rice flour as you would semolina and add puréed fruit for a lovely breakfast. An easier alternative is to pour boiling water on three teaspoons of fine oatmeal and leave to stand for a few minutes. Pureed fruit, mashed banana, yogurt, expressed breast or cow's milk may be added to this. Millet flakes may be bought in health food shops and these can be prepared in the same way as for oatmeal. As the child gets older porridge oats may be used in place of oatmeal and the banana may be sliced instead of mashed.

The importance of chewing

The strongest muscle in the body for its size is the jaw muscle. It needs plenty of exercise right from the start. So babies need banana, whole beans, vegetables that are not puréed but just chopped, pieces of apple, pear or grapes and other foods that need a bit of work as soon as he can handle them. Most chewing is done with molars (the teeth at the back of the mouth) and these do not appear until twelve to twenty-four months, so some foods will be just about impossible. However these teeth are formed and lying in wait just beneath the gums so the baby's jaw will be more effective than an elderly person's jaw which has lost all its teeth.

The importance of milk for calcium

If for any reason a mother is not breastfeeding her baby between the ages of six months and one year it is important to provide a substitute — either cow's milk or soya milk with added dolomite powder (if you cannot get dolomite powder you will need to crush dolomite tablets) which provides calcium and magnesium much needed for bone growth.

There is some evidence that some children who react allergically to cow's milk do not react to goat's milk. However before the age of two years a child should not be given unpasteurized milk.

Don't make your child a sugar addict

Sugar is just as bad for children as it is for adults. They too have to cope with the sudden increase in blood sugar by producing more and more insulin to bring the balance back to normal. If this balance is lost, both physical and mental well-being are, in turn, unbalanced. Low blood glucose (hypoglycaemia) and high blood glucose (hyperglycaemia) can have similar and wide-ranging effects: irritability, aggressive outbursts, nervousness, depression, crying spells, confusion, forgetfulness, inability to concentrate, fatigue, insomnia, headaches, palpitations, muscle cramps, excess sweating, digestive problems, allergies and excessive thirst.

It doesn't take long for a baby or child to learn that sugar can, at least temporarily, relieve these symptoms. Unfortuately, for most people it takes years to learn that sugar helped cause the problem in the first place.

But what can you do to reverse the problem and solve the addiction to sugar? The first step is not to encourage the habit in children. But when all is said and done how do you keep a bear away from honey? For children and adults alike the answer is first to get used to less sweet food. Sweets can be substituted for fruit or the occasional home made fruit bar. 'Desserts' can be replaced with 'starters' or just fruit.

In fact there's good evidence that a large part of the sweet tooth syndrome is a learned habit. This was demonstrated in a study in Israel which compared taste preferences for increasingly sweet sucrose solutions in both city and country dwellers, all twelve year-old boys. The city boys preferred a solution more than twice as sweet, and consequently had far more fillings and tooth decay. Living in Jerusalent they had more access to sweets and had clearly acquired the sugar habit. [57]

Most sugar is hidden

There are many different kinds of sugars, some of which occur naturally in quite high concentrations in healthy foods. Others which are added. Over half our sugar intake comes from snack foods. Just avoiding sugar isn't enough. You also need to check the labels of the food you eat.

Ingredients are listed in order of content size, so the higher sugar is on the list the more the food contains. And sugar means dextrose, sucrose (table sugar), maltose and glucose. On the rare occasion when you need to add some sweetness to a dish, a little honey, molasses or maple syrup is better than sugar. Just sweetening dishes with soaked, dried fruit is better still.

How to keep your baby sugar free
But the best way to keep babies off sugar is to go back to the natural diet and eat lots of fresh fruit. And don't be alarmed if an eighteen month-old baby eats four pieces of fruit a day. Another good habit to encourage is drinking diluted fruit juice and plain water, plain water should be the usual drink, with diluted fruit juice just occasionally. A breastfed baby can go from breast to juice diluted one part juice to four parts water, as well as plain bottled or filtered water. If the child already drinks fruit juices straight, then a slow weaning process is needed, slowly diluting the juice more and more.

Don't use sweets for treats
Sugar addiction has two elements: the body's physical reaction and dependence on it and the psychological 'have a sweet — make it better' syndrome. Just as with training your child to like savoury foods it is most important to work on the psychological element from an early age. The golden rule here is:
Never give sweets, biscuits, cake or fruit as a reward for being good, as something to cheer a child up either after a physical bump or because he/she is just miserable or bored.

Fussiness and food fads
'My child will only eat chocolate yogurt.' 'My child will only eat spaghetti hoops and baked beans.' 'My child will only eat potatoes, carrots and baked beans.' Anyone who has anything to do with children will recognize these phrases well. However, how do these children and their parents get into the situation, how do they get out of it and can it be avoided?

As with any problem prevention is always the easiest form of cure. There are five points to remember in this situation:

1. Provided the diet is balanced young children don't need great variety. While they do prefer sweeter vegetables like carrots to bitter foods they do not have great taste discrimination. Texture is more important to them.

2. If you do not have chocolate yogurt/spaghetti hoops or whatever other junk food these children decide to eat solely then you will never get into this situation as the option isn't there.

3. Ensure that your child has adequate zinc and is therefore able to taste to his or her full capacity.

4. From the very start eating should be a matter of satiating appetite, not something you do for mummy or something you do tidily or cleanly or politely or even for the starving people in Ethiopia (no three year old can grasp the link between the plate of cauliflower cheese in front of him and those starving on the other side of the world). Eating should be an independent thing that the child does for himself as soon as possible using spoon or hands, whichever is easiest.

5. For a small baby texture is usually more important than flavour so be careful to purée properly and try to avoid slimy things altogether.

Supplements for children
According to Dr Roger Williams, often called the founder of the new nutrition, 'The greatest hope for increasing [health and] lifespan can be offered if nutrition — from the time of prenatal development up to old age — is continuously of the highest quality'. Although diet is crucial and the right place to start, every child can benefit from the proper vitamin and mineral supplementation.

When should you start supplementing?
My view is that as soon as a child has stopped receiving the majority of his or her nourishment from the mother's milk, supplementation should start. This preventative approach is nothing unusual. Every child can receive, free of charge,

vitamin drops from the DHSS. Many women are not aware of this and sometimes the form filling required puts others off. For babies on formula milk these drops are designed to be taken in addition to those provided in the formula. The vitamin drops contain vitamin A 2,000iu, vitamin D 400iu, B_1 1mg, B_2 0.4mg, B_3 0.5mg, B_6 0.5mg and vitamin C 50mg.

While this may ensure the basic levels required for these nutrients, many other important nutrients are excluded. Especially important for the growing child are vitamin A to build up strong membranes less permeable to infection; vitamin D to aid the absorption of calcium; B vitamins and vitamin C involved in brain development; calcium and magnesium for healthy bones; zinc to maintain the integrity of RNA and DNA and assist in growth; essential fatty acids because these get incorporated into every cell especially brain cells; and also iron, chromium, selenium and manganese.

The ideal daily intake for these nutrients is shown below, compared to the Recommended Daily Allowances. The third column shows the sort of level of these nutrients that your baby will get from following the recommendations in this book. The final column shows the amounts that even a good diet falls short. These, plus a little more for safety, are the ideal levels for a one year old to supplement.

THE IDEAL DAILY PROGRAMME

Nutrient	RDA	Optimum Level	From Optimum Diet	Minimum Supplemental Level
Vitamins				
A	1,000iu	4,000iu	15,000iu	(4,000iu)
D	400iu	400iu	40iu	400iu
E		20iu	5iu	20iu
C	20mg	200mg	180mg	100mg
B_1 (thiamine)	0.5mg	5mg	1mg	5mg
B_2 (riboflavin)	0.6mg	5mg	1mg	5mg
B_3 (niacin)	7mg	10mg	7mg	5mg
B_5 (pantothenic acid)		10mg	4mg	5mg
B_6 (pyridoxine)		5mg	2mg	5mg
B_{12}		5mcg	1mcg	2mcg
Folic acid		100mcg	200mcg	50mcg
Biotin		150mcg	?	50mcg
Minerals				
Sodium		1,500mg	868mg	
Potassium		3,000mg	3,200mg	
Calcium	600mg	600mg	624mg	300mg
Magnesium		200mg	240mg	150mg
Iron	7mg	7mg	7mg	5mg
Zinc		7mg	5mg	5mg
Chromium		35mcg	?	10mcg
Manganese		1.5mg	?	1mg
Selenium		30mcg	?	10mcg

5.2.2 — *Optimum intake from diet and supplements*

Supplements for children either need to be chewable, liquid or powder. Most manufacturers prefer to make chewable tablets. This is fine, however the taste of vitamins is not too nice so the flavour needs to be disguised. This can be done with natural fruit flavourings and a small amount of fructose which is fruit sugar. However, some manufacturers use artifical flavourings and colourings and large amounts of sugar. Liquid supplements, although appealing, are usually in a sugary syrup and are therefore not ideal. Powders are quite useful although not as easy as chewable supplements.

Adjusting for age

Nutrient needs alter with age, however as long as the child is still growing the extra need for calcium, magnesium, zinc and vitamin D is still there. The chart below shows the ideal intakes of each nutrient from birth to ten.

Are there any dangers with supplementing children?

Children tend to be more susceptible to vitamin toxicity than adults. However, as with all nutrients it is the dosage that counts. The doses listed below are well within any potentially toxic limits for even the most sensitive child and are therefore non-toxic. However, larger doses of vitamin A or D are not recommended in children unless advised by a doctor or nutritionist.

OPTIMUM DAILY INTAKES FROM AGE ONE TO ELEVEN RECOMMENDED BY ION

Nutrient	Age: Less than 1	1	2	3-4	5-6	7-8	9-11
Vitamins							
A	4,000iu	4,500	5,000	5,500	6,000	7,000	7,500
D	400iu	400	400	400	400	400	400
E	20iu	20	25	30	35	45	60
C	100mg	100	200	300	400	500	600
B_1 (thiamine)	5mg	5	6	8	12	16	20
B_2 (riboflavin)	5mg	5	6	8	12	16	20
B_3 (niacin)	7mg	10	14	16	18	20	22
B_5 (pantothenic acid)	10mg	10	15	20	25	30	35
B_6 (pyridoxine)	5mg	5	7	10	12	16	20
B_{12}	5mcg	6	7	8	9	10	10
Folic acid	100mcg	100	120	140	160	180	200
Biotin	150mcg	150	180	210	240	270	300
Minerals							
Sodium	3,000mg	3,000	3,000	3,000	3,000	3,000	3,000
Potassium	3,000mg	3,500	3,750	4,000	4,250	4,500	5,000
Calcium	600mg	600	700	800	900	1,000	1,100
Magnesium	200mg	200	225	250	300	350	375
Iron	7mg	7	8	8	9	10	10
Zinc	7mg	7	8	9	10	12	14
Chromium	35mcg	35	37	40	43	45	50
Manganese	1.5mg	2	2.5	3	3.5	4	4.5
Selenium	30mcg	33	37	40	43	47	50

Chart 5.2.3 — *Optimum supplemented vitamins and minerals by age*

CHAPTER 5.3

Nutrition during pregnancy

—OVERVIEW—

Pregnancy is a time of extremely rapid growth so naturally enough it places considerably increased demands on the mother's nutritional status. However the best time to make any necessary nutritional changes is before conception.

For some people even becoming pregnant can be a problem. Infertility affects one in every four couples to some degree in the UK. For men sperm quantity and mobility are important and vitamin C and zinc can improve both. For women zinc and B_6 are necessary for the sex hormone gonadotrophin.

During pregnancy itself the requirements for a number of nutrients increases. Vitamins B_1, B_2, B_6, B_{12}, folic acid and the minerals zinc, iron, calcium and magnesium are needed in increased amount for growth. A deficiency of any one of them has been linked with abnormality. Folic acid in particular is associated with an increased risk of spina bifida. Too high levels of the toxic minerals lead, cadmium and copper can reduce growth and development and increase the risks of abnormality. All these toxic metals can be lowered by nutritional means so it is good to measure their levels before conception. Hair analysis is the most convenient and accurate form of measurement for lead.

Getting pregnant is a risky business. For example, out of all pregnancies in Britain in 1983, more than 89,000 had problems. 27,000 ended

in miscarriage, there were 6,000 perinatal deaths, 14,000 babies were born with physical defects and 42,000 were low birthweight babies. Roughly one in seven pregnancies go wrong.

The good news is that the large majority of these problems can be totally avoided if the nutrition of the mother is optimum prior to and during pregnancy. Further information on the latest developments in this area can be obtained by sending a sae to Foresight, The Old Vicarage, Church Lane, Witley, Surrey.[58]

Writing in the 1970s Dr Jennings says this:

> It seems that much more could be done in the field of preventive medicine to cut down the large numbers of preventable congenital defects. In human foetal development, most abnormalities are established by the eighth week to tenth week of pregnancy. This means, of course, that the most important period for nutritional care occurs in the few weeks before and immediately after conception.

Pregnancy is something that must be prepared for in advance.

Today, more than ever before, miscarriage is the greatest threat to any pregnancy. One in ten pregnancies end in miscarriage. This figure is likely to be an underestimation since early miscarriages are often not reported — or even go unnoticed. It has been estimated that for every successful conception, there are three early miscarriages, in which the ovum may have been fertilized but failed to implant properly. The woman may notice nothing more than a delayed or missed period, sometimes followed by a heavier period than usual. Once a pregnancy is beyond twenty-eight weeks one in every sixty-five women will lose their baby.

Experts believe that miscarriage is the most sensitive of all indications that a woman or her partner are exposed to environment hazards. Researchers from Columbia University in New York decided to investigate the risk factors associated with miscarriage in 2,802 New York women. They found that the risk of miscarriage increased with consumption of cigarettes and alcohol. A drinker and smoker had a four times higher risk of miscarriage. Those who didn't smoke but had a drink every day still had a risk more than two and a half times higher than the abstainer. Certainly the most widely used poison for the unborn child is alcohol.

The foetal alcohol syndrome

Miscarriage may be nature's way of terminating a pregnancy that was destined to go wrong, but many babies are born suffering from the effects of maternal alcohol consumption. The signs and symptoms, now well documented, are known as foetal alcohol syndrome. 'Its main signs are low birth weight and mild facial deformity' according to a report in the New Scientist in August 1985.

The flattened midface, often with a thin upper lip, is connected to a short nose with little nostril flare. The eyelid openings are short, the ears often misshapen, and the lower jaw long. Many affected babies also have heart murmurs, persistent ear infections leading to deafness, droopy eyelids, squint, congenital hip dislocations, and fingers and toes that may be short, partly fused, angled, lacking in flexion, and with small nails.

These are the most commonly physical abnormalities resulting from alcohol in pregnancy.

Alcohol also affects mental development and behaviour too. Victims of foetal alcohol syndrome are often hyperactive, jittery and have difficulty sleeping. But a baby doesn't have to have the physical signs to be mentally defected by alcohol, according to Canadian researchers at Queens University in Ontario. They investigated whether there was any difference in mental development in children whose mothers drank or smoked at socially accepted levels during pregnancy. They found that verbal skills, both in speaking and understanding, were poorer in the children from these mothers.

How much is too much?

His views are backed up by the recent Columbia University study which showed that even the consumption of a single drink every other day increased the risk of miscarriage. Profesor David Smith from Washington, recognized as a world authority on foetal alcohol syndrome, points out that 'there is no known teratogen yet studied in man which clearly shows a threshold effect where the substance is quite safe to a particular level, beyond which it is teratogenic'.

Many environmental hazards, including alcohol, are at their most dangerous at the very early stages of pregnancy, when cell division is at its highest. So alcohol really needs to be avoided from the time a couple choose to get pregnant, not just when the woman discovers she is.

But it isn't only the woman who needs to abstain. Alcohol damages sperm, and at least in animals, alcohol consumption in the male does result in a greater risk for birth defects and miscarriage in future children.

Alcohol the anti-nutrient

Alcohol is the best example of a substance that may do its damage by compromising good nutrition. As well as affecting absorption of nutrients, it interferes with their positive health action in body chemistry. Nutrients like B_6, iron and zinc, so badly needed during pregnancy, are badly affected when alcohol is drunk in excess. This leads to greater needs for B_6 which are higher anyway during pregnancy.

Most of all, alcohol consumption badly affects the availability of zinc, so crucial for pregnancy. Research at Oregon State University has revealed that consumption of alcohol while on a zinc sufficient diet produces zinc deficiency, equivalent to that of a zinc deficient diet without any extra alcohol. So alcohol is a powerful anti-zinc factor during gestation and lactation.[59]

Cigarettes and pregnancy

Smoking in pregnancy reduces birthweight, affects mental development of the child in later years and provides an increased risk of cancer to both mother and baby.

The Royal College of Physicians' report 'Health and Smoking' concludes:

> Women who smoke are more likely to be infertile or take longer to conceive than women who do not smoke. Smokers who become pregnant have a small increase in the risk of spontaneous abortion, bleeding during pregnancy and the development of various placental abnormalities.

But most marked of all is the incidence of low birthweight babies among smoking mothers.

This effect on birth size is caused by cigarette smoke's ability to slow down the rate of growth of the foetus. It may do this by damaging the DNA, our blueprint for survival. This in turn has far more serious consequences for mental and physical development. These consequences include a greater risk of having a premature baby, a reduced ability to ward off infection for the young infant and lower mental development.

Smoking lowers intelligence

The effects of maternal smoking can be seen many years later in the child. A massive survey at Pennsylvania State University involving 9,024 children looked at differences between children who were born to mothers who smoked during pregnancy compared to children of the same mothers when the mother didn't smoke during pregnancy. 'This study confirms reports that children of women who smoked cigarettes throughout pregnancy have small impairments in intelligence and increased frequencies of short attention span and hyperactive behaviour.'[60]

Smoking increases illnesses in children

An important concept in nutrition today is that of 'organ reserve'. It's like being born with £100 in the bank. As each organ is taxed the bank balance drops. Eventually the organ will malfunction, but before that, the reserve that organ has before malfunction occurs may already have diminished substantially. People with low organ reserve may function well until their body is subjected to stress. Those with weak immune systems are more susceptible to infections. Those with poor hormone and nerve balance succumb to the ravages of stress. Children born to mothers who smoke appear to have an overall poor organ reserve as illustrated by their greater susceptibility to illness. Dr Rantakallio compared frequency of illness in children of smokers or non-smokers and found a 43% increase in illnesses among the smokers' children. These included more blood disorders, more respiratory infections, more bladder and kidney problems and more skin disorders.[61]

Preventing sickness in pregnancy

During the first three months of pregnancy all the organs of the baby are completely formed. It is during this period — and of course, before conception, that optimum nutrition is most important. Yet many women experience continual sickness and don't feel like eating healthily.

Misnamed as 'morning' sickness, this condition has been accepted as normal during the early part of pregnancy. Up to 70% of women experience pregnancy sickness, some for as little as a week, others for the entire pregnancy. The most common signs and symptoms are nausea, usually worse on an empty stomach, and often triggered by smells of certain foods or perfumes; retching first thing in the morning or before meals; vomiting after eating; aversions to some foods and cravings for others; a metallic taste in the mouth; a feeling of hunger even when feeling nauseous; and relief from nausea by eating.

Pregnancy sickness is one example of a condition which usually only manifests in women whose nutritional status is less than optimum. Probably caused by increase in a hormone called 'human chorionic gonadotrophin', women with poor diets are particularly at risk. This hormone, HCG for short, is produced by the developing placenta from the moment of conception. It usually reaches its peak around nine to ten weeks after the last period, and declines by week fourteen to sixteen. Although it is produced later in pregnancy, the quantities present are far less. In very undernourished mothers HCG may not be produced in sufficient quantities at all, which may explain why women who miscarry early in pregnancy are less likely to experience any pregnancy sickness. On the other hand, very well nourished women appear to ride the storm of these hormonal changes with little or no symptoms of nausea at all.

Other possible explanations for nausea or sickness involve the body trying to eliminate toxins, and also difficulty maintaining blood sugar balance. Blood sugar levels control your appetite and at night, after many hours without eating, blood sugar levels reach their lowest. Many women find that eating little and often helps to reduce the experience of nausea.

Diet to prevent pregnancy sickness

Ensure that you get enough complex carbohydrates, which includes beans, lentils, vegetables and whole grains like brown rice. As these are not the easiest foods to snack on, they are best eaten as part of major meals, relying on fruit and seeds, like sunflower seeds for snacks. The real keys to avoiding pregnancy sickness are:

- Always eat breakfast, preferably containing some protein foods, like yogurt or eggs.
- Eat small meals and frequent snacks of fruit and seeds. There is no limit to how much fresh fruit you can eat in a day.
- Avoid all sugar and refined foods.
- Avoid high fat 'junk' food, containing long lists of additives and preservatives.
- Decrease your intake of dried fruit or undiluted fruit juice, both of which provided concentrated sugar.
- Drink plenty of water between meals.
- Avoid or decrease your intake of coffee and tea.
- Avoid all alcohol and cigarettes.

During pregnancy the need for vitamin B_6, B_{12}, folic acid, iron and zinc all increase and extra supplements of these usually stop even the worst cases of pregnancy sickness. Vitamin B_6 is poorly supplied in the average diet. The RDA for B_6 in America is 2mg and most of us get less than this. However, during pregnancy minimal needs are at least 3mg and often 100mg are needed to stop pregnancy sickness. The recommended therapeutic dose of B_{12} and folic acid respectively is 250mcg and 400mcg. Normally, symptoms will disappear within two weeks, at which point these doses can be halved.

The mineral zinc may also be implicated in pregnant women who feel nauseous and go off food. According to Dr Pfeiffer and Mrs Barnes of the Foresight organization for pre-conceptual care:

> The nauseated woman is usually deficient in both zinc and B_6. Both are needed for growing tissues of any kind and the foetus and uterus make extraordinary demands on the mother's supply. Vitamin B_6 has been used for nausea and vomiting of pregnancy with some success. We have had many pregnant patients who had difficulties with previous pregnancies go through a pregnancy on a zinc and B_6 regime with no difficulties.

The minimum need for zinc during pregnancy is 20mg a day while the average diet supplies less than 10mg. So zinc supplementation is a must during pregnancy and doubly important if you experience nausea.[62]

Preventing problems of pregnancy

There are a number of minor health problems that can and frequently do occur in pregnancy. Some of these can be prevented or alleviated with nutrition.

Anaemia

Mild anaemia may be present in one in three pregnant women. The symptoms include pallor, tiredness, a sore tongue and a feeling almost as if there's a weight on your shoulders. It is usually the result of a low level of iron in the blood protein haemoglobin, however B_{12}, folic acid, manganese and B_6 deficiency can also result in anaemia. Supplementing 20mg of iron in the ferrous not ferric form, for example ferrous sulphate, should alleviate this problem Occasionally 40mg may be required. B_{12} deficiency anaemia is called pernicious anaemia. The symptoms of this can be masked by supplementing folic acid, so if folic acid is supplemented B_{12} needs to be taken as well.

Constipation

Many imagine their abdominal organs — stomach, liver, pancreas, bladder and intestines — to live in spacious surroundings. Actually they are closely packed together. The arrival of a baby plus placenta, enlarged uterus and fluid, is a very tight fit and results in less room for the intestines, stomach and bladder to expand. For many women this means a greater chance for constipation since the faecal matter in the large intestine is more compressed and the muscles have less room to keep the contents moving along. The answer is not to take laxatives, but to make sure your diet is especially high in fluids and fibre and low in mucus-forming foods. Dairy produce, eggs and meat are especially mucus forming and tend to make faecal matter more compacted and harder to pass along. On the other hand, fruits, vegetables, grains, lentils and beans are high in fibre and this fibre absorbs fluid, making the resulting faecal matter light and bulky and easier to pass. It is a good idea to drink about a pint of water a day, either as it is or in diluted fruit juice. While this amount of water isn't strictly needed to maintain the water balance of the body it does help relieve constipation.

Eclampsia and pre-eclampsia

Eclampsia is a disease that only occurs in pregnancy. The first early warning sign of pre-eclampsia is raised blood-pressure. The blood pressure may be only slightly raised to 140/90. This may be accompanied by slight oedema in ankles and protein in the urine. It is quite common, occurring in 5% of pregnancies. Once the pregnancy is over the symptoms all go away. However, eclampsia can be very serious indeed causing fits which can endanger the life of the mother and baby. It is for this reason that regular

check-ups are very important since women with pre-eclampsia don't necessarily feel ill.

The condition is thought to be connected with incomplete formation of the placenta. The placenta keeps mother's and baby's blood supply separate, preventing the mother's immune system reacting to the 'foreign body' as it would to a virus or cancer cell. This mechanism may be at fault due to a malformed placenta. The larger the baby becomes the less well this poorly functioning system can manage, which is why pre-eclampsia occurs towards the end of a pregnancy. Mothers who have had pre-eclampsia in the first child are usually much better in the second. This is thought to be due to an adaptation of the immune system. According to medical researchers Ylastalo and Ylikorkala, the exaggerated rise in copper may also be a factor in pre-eclamptic toxaemia.[63]

Hypertension

This is unlikely to occur in those who have had no previous history of high blood-pressure. If the blood-pressure rises above 160/100 the person must be carefully monitored. This is usually accompanied by oedema (fluid retention) in face, hands, ankles and abdomen. There is no known medical cure, although bed rest often helps. Drugs are avoided where possible since these can affect the supply of blood to the baby. The nutritional recommendations mentioned for pre-eclampsia are applicable here too.

Leg cramps

Cramps are almost invariably caused by an imbalance of calcium and magnesium. These minerals, as well as sodium and potassium, are called electrolytes because they control the electrical balance that turns muscle cells on and off. Cramps are caused by muscles going into contraction. Deficiency of calcium, magnesium or sodium can cause this, however sodium deficiency is extremely rare. Because of the baby's demand for calcium and magnesium to make healthy bones, pregnant women often become deficient. While milk products are particularly high in calcium they are almost complete devoid of magnesium. Green leafy vegetables, nuts and seeds are quite good sources of both calcium and magnesium. However, eating more of these foods often doesn't provide enough calcium and magnesium to banish cramps completely. A dietary supplement of Dolomite, which is calcium and magnesium, is therefore advisable.

Stretch marks

The skin on the abdomen does a remarkable stretching job in pregnancy. If the skin loses its natural elasticity stretch marks may develop. Stretch marks on the stomach, thighs, breasts, hips or shoulder girdle are one of the signs of zinc deficiency so adequate zinc intake is crucial. Vitamin C is needed to make collagen, the inter-cellular glue, and vitamin E helps to keep skin supple. Applying vitamin E oil or cream is helpful during the last weeks of pregnancy and after the birth to encourage the skin to contract. Most of all, abdominal muscles must be kept strong throughout pregnancy and afterwards otherwise you will be left with a flabby tummy. It takes many months to return abdominal muscles to their former strength and regular abdominal exercises after pregnancy are essential.

Varicose veins

The development of varicose veins during pregnancy is not at all uncommon. This is caused by the restricted flow of blood returning from the feet and legs in the groin area due to the baby and also due to constipation. All the blood vessels in the legs lead to one big vein in the groin. If this is compressed the blood must return along different routes. this can cause small veins on the surface of the legs to become enlarged. The result is prominent veins that have lost their elasticity and are no longer able to maintain proper blood flow.

The secret of avoiding these unsightly blood vessels is to keep the veins in good shape and to minimize the restriction of blood flow. Vitamin C is needed to make collagen which keeps the arteries supple. Vitamin B_3 helps to dilate the blood vessels, while vitamin E and the essential fatty acid EPA (high in fish) thin the blood and help to transports oxygen in the blood. A high fibre diet helps to reduce constipation, removing additional pressure on the main vein in the groin

ara, and regular exercise helps to stimulate proper circulation.

A better diet for pregnancy

Even if your diet is perfectly adequate when you're not pregnant there's no reason to assume it is adequate when you are. At any time of stress, which includes puberty, menopause, menstruation, but most of all pregnancy, nutritional needs are greatest.

The protein myth

During pregnancy protein is used more efficiently. Most of our protein is used to make cells that we're made of. The excess gets converted into energy. In pregnancy less protein is used for energy and more is stored for use by the baby. For this reason urea levels in the blood, which are an indication of protein breakdown, often drop in pregnancy. This protein storing means that the need for increased protein is spread over the entire pregnancy.

The recommended intake for protein goes up 11% in pregnancy. On top of the normal protein requirement of 54g we need an extra 6g a day maximum. Some nutritionists consider that this estimate is too high. The overall need for protein depends on both the quality of the protein and the dietary intake of vitamins and minerals which determines how well you use protein . So if you eat good quality protein and are not vitamin or mineral deficient you can afford to eat less than this. The absolute minimum requirement for protein during pregnancy is 49g a day.

No sugar thanks

Probably the most important dietary change in pregnancy is to cut down on sugar. Not only is sugar bad for you and your baby but also most sources of sugar are what the nutritionists call 'empty calories' — they supply the calories but no nutrients to go with it. As much as two-thirds of most people's calorie intake is from empty-calorie foods consisting of refined sugars and fat.

Very high levels of sugar in the form of glucose interfere with normal sugar metabolism, and can cause birth defects. The same effects do not appear with fructose or galactose which are the forms of sugar found in fruit and dairy produce. So if you have an uncontrollable sweet tooth eat lots of fruit instead.

During pregnancy many women become mildly hypoglycaemic. This means their blood sugar level fluctuates abnormally. They learn that eating sugary foods, or having another coffee (which causes the mobilization of sugar from the liver) makes them feel temporarily better. But 'temporarily' is the key word. Any regular over-consumption of sugar, alcohol, strong tea or coffee can lead to ever-worsening signs of hypoglycaemia.

Fibre

One of the difficulties most often encountered during pregnancy is constipation. Later on in pregnancy the baby will press on the stomach and intestines, making it harder to eat a lot and making you prone to constipation. In pregnancy a high fibre diet is doubly important. But this doesn't mean just adding bran to a fibre poor diet. It is far better to get your fibre from the foods you eat. All vegetables, grains, nuts, lentils and beans contain significant amounts of fibre.

Supplements during pregnancy

Some doctors warn against vitamin and mineral supplementation during pregnancy. Among those who are unfamiliar with nutrition there is a belief that one needs to be extremely careful with pregnant women and children. This of course is true. However, the best care possible is to ensure adequate nutrient intake and to minimize exposure to pollutants and unnecessary medication. Iron and folic acid supplements are frequently given to pregnant women without testing if they are needed.

But on the other hand, we estimate that only five in a hundred women during pregnancy have a diet that meets all the recommended daily allowances. This is why supplementation is not only a wise precaution but is a definite must in pregnancy, providing it is properly supervised.

It is well established that nutritional deficiency in animals will cause birth abnormalities. This has been shown with B_2, B_3, B_5 (pantothenic acid), B_6 and folic acid. To ensure optimum nutrition in pregnancy it is necessary to take some vitamin and mineral supplements even if your diet is well balanced in other respects. However there are some vitamins which should not be taken in large amounts during pregnancy. One of these is vitamin A.

The dangers of taking too much vitamin A

Vitamin A is a fat soluble vitamin found in foods of animal origin and particularly in liver, since this is where it stores in the body. Cod liver oil is a popular source for vitamin A although it can also be made synthetically. Some synthetic forms of vitamin A are far more toxic than the natural vitamin A and it is these that have caused great concern recently.

Vitamin A is vital for proper foetal growth and plays an important part in visual development. The RDA for pregnant women is 2,250iu and the optimum level anywhere between 7,500iu and 15,000iu. However, in the view of the somewhat exaggerated reports of vitamin A toxicity it is wise not to take any more than this unless you have clear deficiency symptoms and are under the supervision of a doctor or nutritionist.

Vitamin D is vital for healthy bones

Unlike any other vitamin, vitamin D can be made in the skin in the presence of sunlight. Vitamin D deficiency is not common in Britain, except in pregnant Asian women, who for reasons of skin colour, filter out the sun's ultraviolet rays and produce less vitamin D. However, although vitamin D deficiency is not good news for the mother, some evidence suggests that the baby is not greatly affected. In one study the babies of forty-five Asian women, nineteen of which had received supplements of 1,000iu of vitamin D, and twelve white women were compared for mineralization of bones. None of the children showed any abnormal level of bone mineralization.

Cauliflowers and vitamin K

Vitamin K is called the clotting factor because it is involved in the manufacture of prothrombin, which makes your blood clot. Normally it is manufactured by bacteria in the gut. However, a baby's gut is sterile after birth and must rely on the mother's supply. Breast milk contains a factor that inhibits vitamin K so breast feeding mothers need to take special care to eat enough cauliflower and cabbage which are high in vitamin K. Unexplained bleeding in young infants can be due to vitamin K deficiency. Fortunately vitamin K deficiency is extremely rare and usually only occurs in people with known digestive disorders that impair absorption of nutrients.

All B vitamins are needed during pregnancy, however only the need for B_6, B_{12}, folic acid and biotin increase substantially.

B_6 and pregnancy

Britain has no recommended levels for B_6. In America 2mg is recommended daily, and extrapolated from this figure (based on a pregnant woman's increased need for protein, which B_6 helps to metabolize) the RDA for a pregnant woman is 2.6mg. But this simply isn't enough to maintain normal biochemical functions. B_6 levels in the blood decline rapidly during pregnancy dropping from 11.3mcg/ml by the end, strongly implying B_6 depletion. Studies have also shown decreased B_6 dependent enzyme activity until people are given at least 7.5mg on top of the average deficient diet which supplies less than 1.5mg. So that's 9mg in all just to prevent obvious deficiency. The optimum level for B_6 is probably between 25 and 100mg, and more likely 50 to 100mg during pregnancy and breastfeeding.

B_{12} and folic acid

Vitamin B_{12} and folic acid are particularly important in pregnancy. Normal foetal development depends upon these nutrients. One of the indications of the importance of B_{12} is the fact that the levels found in newborn babies are more than twice that found in the mother. Adequate B_{12} nutrition also appears to increase the uptake of folic acid.

The (US) RDA for folic acid is 800mcg during pregnancy. the average intake is about 200mcg,

so the average woman falls a long way short of what is needed. In fact, the World Health Organization reports that from one half to one third of expectant mothers suffer from folic acid deficiency in the last three months of pregnancy. Folic acid in food can be lost by storing or cooking. Folic acid is needed to manufacture DNA and with B_{12} helps to make red blood cells. Folic acid deficiency can produce irritability, sluggishness, forgetfulness and cheilosis (a condition characterized by lesions at the side of the mouth). But the most significant symptom of deficiency in pregnancy is pernicious anaemia. According to Dr Pfeiffer 'Many women with a history of abortion and miscarriage have been able to complete successful childbirth subsequent to folic acid supplementation.' It is now generally thought that a folic acid supplement of at least 300mcg should be taken to minimize the risk of deficiency.

Biotin

This vital B vitamin is often excluded in popular A to Z's of vitamins, yet its role in pregnancy is of the greatest important. Biotin is needed to make fatty acids and most of all is needed to ensure that B_{12} and folic acid are used properly. The normal recommended intake is 150mcg to 300mcg. Probably 300mcg represents an ideal intake during pregnancy.

Vitamin C

Vitamin C has so many roles in pregnancy it's hard to know where to start. It helps make collagen the intercellular glue that keeps skin supple and is therefore vital for preventing stretch marks. It helps to carry oxygen to every cell, nourishing the baby, and builds a strong infection fighting system, keeping the mother in good form. Its need goes up in pregnancy and a daily intake of 2,000mg is recommended.

Vitamin E

Like vitamin C, E helps get oxygen to the cells and protects the vital RNA and DNA from damage which could result in congenital defects in the baby. It also speeds up wound healing and helps to keep skin supple. It is particularly useful if applied externally for those who give birth by Caesarian section. I have seen scars completely disappear with application of vitamin E. The optimum level in pregnancy is 400iu per day.

Minerals for the healthy mother

Just as important as vitamins, and perhaps even more frequently deficient, are the trace minerals. 'Trace element deficiencies and imbalances due to a multitude of causes may be an underlying problem in many cases of neonatal death, congenital anomaly and disorders of pregnancy, as well as poor childhood development', according to nutritionist Elizabeth Lodge Rees writing in *Trace Elements in Health*. While we are very aware of the need for extra iron, what about the lesser known trace elements zinc, manganese, chromium or selenium?[64]

Iron deficiency is common

Iron deficiency is very common in pregnancy. As many as 32% of women may show milk iron deficiency anaemia in pregnancy, with symptoms of lethargy, pale skin and a sore tongue. For this reason doctors always test the haemoglobin level in the blood. Haemoglobin is a protein containing iron that carries oxygen to every cell in the body. Haemoglobin levels frequently fall below 12.6g/dl at which point some iron should be supplemented, or if the diet is low, this should be corrected.

The RDA for iron is 12mg in the UK and 18mg in the USA. Rarely more than 25mg is needed. However pregnant women are often prescribed 180mg or more. This is far too much and interferes with the absorption of other minerals. Iron absorption from non-haem sources is considerably enhanced by vitamin C so eating vitamin C rich foods helps.

Calcium and magnesium

Calcium, phosphorus and magnesium are the major minerals in the human body. Most of this is in the bones and as such the pregnant woman needs a lot more than usual for the baby to build healthy bones. The normal requirement for calcium is 500mg. In a survey released in 1986 it was found that 73% of women get less than 500mg of calcium.[65] The requirement for calcium in pregnancy is 1,200mg per day. That's almost three times more than the average intake and quite frankly it's just about impossible to get without supplementing. Green leafy vegetables, nuts and seeds are high in calcium and magnesium. Many diet textbooks recommend mothers to drink half a litre of milk which supplies 600mg of calcium, but not much magnesium.

Dolomite is the best type of calcium to supplement since it contains magnesium in the right balance. Some dolomite supplements contain extra vitamin D, which is needed to ensure proper absorption of calcium.

Magnesium is not only needed for healthy bones but according to Belinda Barnes of Foresight 'Rats fed a magnesium deficient diet give birth to smaller rats with more congenital malformations'. Most of the population in Britain are also fed a magnesium deficient diet. The US RDA is 450mg during pregnancy, but the average daily intake is only 249mg.

Zinc and foetal growth

The supplementation of zinc is of paramount importance in pregnancy. A pregnant woman needs at least 20mg a day and frequently gets less than half of this from her diet. There are more grounds for supplementing zinc in pregnancy than any other mineral. Zinc is involved in about 100 different enzyme reactions in the body, many of which are involved in growth. And it is during times of greatest growth (pregnancy, puberty, wound healing) that zinc deficiency can wreak havoc. In fact, zinc deficiency is associated with genetic abnormalities, because DNA and RNA, which hold the 'blueprint' for our cells, can't function without zinc. Low levels of zinc are found in stillborn babies and even potential fathers become infertile without it.

But what is new and vitally important is the startling research findings of Professor Bryce-Smith on so called 'normal' mothers and babies. After some initial discoveries that high lead and cadmium levels and low zinc were associated with stillbirths, difficult pregnancies and deformed babies, it was imperative to launch a comprehensive study to determine just how important these minerals are. So in 1980 Professor Bryce-Smith set out to test no less than thirty-six different minerals in a dozen different ways, both in mothers and babies. He measured hair levels, blood levels, amniotic fluid, placental levels, pubic hair, cord blood . . . you name it, he tested it! The first question he asked was 'What is normal?' and to find this out he selected 100 normal births, producing normal babies. Much to his surprise, their mineral levels were far from normal. He found that the lower the zinc levels in placenta, the higher the lead and cadmium levels, the smaller was the baby.[66]

Copper *vs* zinc

Zinc and copper are well known enemies so zinc needs to go up if copper is in excess. Although copper levels rise in pregnancy and too much can be dangerous, too little is not a good idea either. In animals copper deficiency has been shown to cause cell structure changes in the aorta. A good wholefood diet with plenty of beans and lentils will provide enough copper. If supplements are taken no more than 1mg a day should be taken with at least 15mg of zinc, since copper and zinc compete. However one of the top experts in trace elements Dr Carl Pfeiffer, believes there are hardly ever good grounds for supplementing copper at all.

At the Brain Bio Center we have determined serum copper in more than 12,000 patients and have not found a single case of copper deficiency. Foetal liver at term contains approximately seven times the concentration of copper found normally in adult liver. Five to fifteen years are needed to bring this down. Levels of copper in the blood are elevated by

Nutrient	Optimum level	Optimum dietary intake	Recommended supplemental level
Vitamins			
A	7,500iu	25,000iu	(max 10,000iu)
D	400iu	200iu	200iu
E	400iu	20iu	380iu
C	1,500mg	200mg	1,800mg
B_1 (thiamine)	25mg	2mg	23mg
B_2 (riboflavin)	25mg	3mg	23mg
B_3 (niacin)	50mg	25mg	25mg
B_5 (pantothenic acid)	50mg	30mg	20mg
B_6 (pyridoxine)	100mg	21mg	79mg
B_{12}	50mcg	15mcg	25mcg
Folic acid	800mcg	600mcg	200mcg
Biotin	200mcg	?	100mcg
Minerals			
Sodium	3,000mg	2,000mg	
Potassium	5,000mg	6,000mg	
Calcium	1,200mg	1,500mg	(max 800mg)
Magnesium	600mg	600mg	(max 300mg)
Iron	18mg	25mg	(max 20mg)
Zinc	20mg	10mg	10mg
Chromium	50mcg	?30mcg	20mcg
Manganese	5mg	?3mg	2mg
Selenium	25mcg	?15mcg	10mcg

Chart 5.3.1 — *Nutritional needs during pregnancy*

oestrogens; therefore levels of copper rise progressively during pregnancy. Serum copper is normally 115mg/dl at conception and rises to 260mg/dl at term.

Supplements for a healthy pregnancy

The chart on the previous page shows the optimum levels of nutrients in pregnancy that we work to at the Institute for Optimum Nutrition (ION) with supplementation. Some of these are the same as the RDAs and some are a lot higher. The next column shows the levels that an optimum diet alone could supply. The final column **Recommended Supplemental Level** represents what one would need to supplement to reach the optimum levels, given that you are eating a well balanced diet.

CHAPTER 5.4

Nutrition and exercise

—OVERVIEW—

Nutrient needs vary substantially from person to person depending on their level of fitness and frequency of exercise. Exercise stimulates metabolism, both demanding more nutrients and improving the overall efficiency of the human body. This increased efficiency, coupled with exercise's effect on improving appetite control, leads to better control of body weight. Exercise is also associated with a decreased risk of cardiovascular disease, diabetes, depression and obesity.

The physical benefits of exercise can be divided into three factors: strength, suppleness and stamina. Different types of exercise develop these qualities to different degrees. They also make differing nutritional demands on the body. Exercises which develop stamina have the most all-round benefits on health, by improving the cardiovascular system and hence the ability to transport oxygen. However, the best forms of exercise, for example swimming, develop all three qualities of strength, suppleness and stamina.

Exercise and good nutrition are closely related not only because both provide positive health benefits, but also because one seems to lead to the other. When interviewed, participants in The Fun Run, an event sponsored by the *Sunday Times* to encourage groups of people to take up jogging, reported eating more wholefoods even though they had not been prompted to do so. In a survey of clients consulting nutritionists at

ION 58% of subjects reported an increased level of exercise. It is, of course, hard to determine whether such increases in exercise are the result of increased energy due to nutritional changes or other factors. An individual making positive changes in eating habits may decide to also improve physical fitness. However 87% of those clients surveyed who reported increased exercise also reported increased energy levels strongly linking these two factors. [67]

Exercise and obesity

The good news about exercise is that you really don't have to be fanatically fit to lose weight. And the reason why is not calories, it's metabolism.

According to the calorie theory, exercise doesn't do much to promote weight loss. After all, a three mile run only burns up 300 calories. That's equivalent to two slices of toast or a piece of apple pie. But this argument, upon which has hinged the preference to eat less rather than exercise more to lose weight, misses four important facts.

The first is that the effects of exercise are cumulative. Running a mile a day only burns up 300 calories, but if you do that three days a week for a year that's 22,000 calories, equivalent to a weight loss of 11 pounds! Also, the amount of calories you burn up depends upon how fit you are to start with, how hard and how long you exercise and how much of you is fat or muscle. For example, consider someone who weighs 14 stone compared to someone weighing 9 stone. If the 14 stone person runs one mile in 8 minutes, and the 9 stone person does it in 10 minutes, the heavier person will use up over

exercises like swimming, jogging or cycling are more aerobic than stop-go exercises like tennis or squash. Exercises like squash are more 'fast-

Energy expenditure during a one hour run (in calories)							
Body weight	MPH	5	6	7	8	9	10
8 stone		405	493	573	655	737	900
9 stone		469	551	643	735	827	920
10 stone		510	611	713	815	917	1020
11 stone		563	675	788	900	1013	1127
12 stone		614	735	858	981	1104	1228
13 stone		663	794	927	1060	1161	1326
14 stone		713	854	997	1139	1282	1426
15 stone		768	919	1074	1227	1381	1536
16 stone		818	980	1143	1307	1471	1675

Chart 5.4.1 — *Energy expenditure during a one hour run*
(Adapted from McArdle, W.D. *et al.*, *Exercise Physiology: Energy, Nutrition and Human Performance.* Lea and Febiger, 1981)

1,000 calories, The chart above shows how many calories you can use up by running, depending on your weight, distance and speed.

An 8 stone person running at five miles per hour for one hour will use up 405 kcals, while a 16 stone person running at 10 miles per hour will use up 1,635 kcals — over three times as much.

Exercise doesn't create instant weight loss

But if you are overfat and underfit to start with, don't expect immediate results through exercise. The reason is this. Most of us are relatively fit in our school years. School encourages us to play sports and children and adolescents are naturally more physically active. Consequently a larger proportion of younger people is muscle rather than fat. Muscle cells need lots of fuel and therefore burn lots of calories. The leaner the muscle gets the more it needs oxygen. The best kind of exercise are 'aerobic' exercises, which means exercises which supply oxygen. In fact, you can measure how hard a muscle is working by how much oxygen it uses up. Continuous

twitch' muscle which uses glucose as fuel. Running uses more 'slow twitch' muscle which uses fat for fuel. You will lose weight playing squash but you have to play it for a long, long time compared to swimming, running or cycling.

So what happens when you leave school, start driving to work rather than walking, and generally cut down your overall amount of physical activity?

First of all, your good lean muscles start to turn to fat. If you go on a crash diet, your body will break down these good lean muscles as well as body fat to use for energy, and in both cases the result is less muscle. And since muscle uses up calories there is less of you to burn up the food you eat. So putting on weight becomes easier.

As you start to exercise you will begin to replace fatty muscle with lean muscle and rebuild muscle that you didn't have before. With extra muscle you'll begin to burn off that excess fat faster and faster. So even though you may not lose weight with exercise to begin with you are replacing fat with muscle and becoming less fat, and that's what counts for long term weight loss.

Housework won't keep you fit

Another myth about exercise is that you can keep fit through housework. Old textbooks will tell you that the average houseperson or sedentary worker will burn up 2,500 calories, so by putting people on a 1,750 calorie diet, the net effect should be a substantial weight loss. But new research and improved methods for measuring energy expenditure show that these figures are slight distortions of the truth. In fact, a sedentary worker or houseperson will burn up around 2,000 calories a day. Reducing intake to 1,750 calories a day would not have a substantial effect.

However, relatively small increases in activity do have an effect on weight loss, if sustained. For example, one study examined the effects of walking on six overfat and underfit young men. Five days a week for sixteen weeks they walked for 90 minutes a day. That's the equivalent of 45 minutes to work and back. They lost an average of 12.5lbs, their percentage of body fat dropped from 23.5% to 18.6% and their blood fat levels improved, which is a measure of heart health. [68]

Unfanatical fitness decreases your appetite

Contrary to popular belief, moderate exercise actually decreases your appetite. According to new evidence on appetite research, both animals and man consistently show decreased appetite with small increases in physical activity. One study looked at an industrial population in West Bengal, India. Those doing sedentary work ate more and consequently weighed more than those doing light work. As the level of work increased from light to heavy workers ate more, but not relative to their energy output. The result was that the heavier the work the lighter the worker. [69]

Job classification	Daily calorie intake (kcal)	Body weight (lbs)
Sedentary	3,300	148
Light work	2,600	118
Medium work	2,800	114
Heavy work	3,400	113
Very heavy work	3,600	113

Chart 5.4.2 — *Effect of exercise*

It appears that a degree of physical activity is necessary for appetite mechanisms to work properly. Those who do not exercise have exaggerated appetites and hence the pounds gradually creep on. With moderate exercise and the other key factors within the Metabolic Diet, there is no need to go hungry while losing weight.

Exercise boosts your metabolic rate

But the most important reason why exercise is a key to weight loss is its effect on your metabolic rate. According to Professor McArdle, exercise physiologist at City University, New York

> Most people can generate metabolic rates that are eight to ten times above the resting value during sustained running, cycling or swimming. Complementing this increased metabolic rate is the observation that vigorous exercise will raise the metabolic rate for up to fifteen hours after exercise.

In fact, other studies have shown that metabolic rate is raised by 25% for fifteen hours and by 10% for forty-eight hours. According to sports physiologist Professor Fenton

> Exercise has a stimulating effect on metabolism which persists throughout the day, raising metabolic rate and leading to the loss of appreciably more fat than would have been predicted for the exercise taken.

The metabolic effect of exercise is far more significant than the calories used up in the exercise itself. Simply by doing 12 minutes of aerobic exercise a day you can substantially increase your metabolic rate, without increasing your appetite. The net result is weight loss.

Exercise, pulse and blood pressure

Exercises which develop stamina also improve the health of the heart and cardiovascular system. The strength of the heart is reflected by your pulse rate. A strong heart may need to beat 60 or less times in a minute to keep the blood flowing around the body. Most people's pulse rate is more than 70 beats per minutes. This decreases with regular exercise.

Blood pressure also decreases with exercise. Since regular exercise lowers triglyceride levels in the blood, this is probably due to a decrease in rate of atherosclerosis.

Increased need for nutrients

All exercise increases the body's demand for nutrients. The primary nutrients are glucose and oxygen from which energy for the muscles is derived. However the release of the energy within glucose and its combination with oxygen require many vitamins and minerals. These are B_1, B_2, B_3 B_5 (pantothenic acid) and vitamin C. The muscles need adequate calcium and magnesium to work. Iron helps transport oxygen, and chromium helps transport glucose. All these nutrients must be adequately supplied to ensure maximum physical performance.

In endurance sports like marathons or triathlons, the short term supplies of glucose and glycogen become used up. The body must therefore turn to fat and protein as sources of fuel. Their metabolism is less energy efficient and it is at this point that athletes are said to 'hit the wall' because they experience a diminished physical output. The conversion of protein and fat to acetyl co-enzyme A, which can then be 'burnt' to produce energy, involves vitamin B_6 and biotin.

Nutrients for more muscle

Muscle is 22% protein. Strength developing exercises encourage the body to build muscle. So it is logical to presume that the more protein you eat the greater the chances of putting on muscle. But this is a myth. Eating extra protein, or taking protein powders, can only build a fraction more muscle even in the most dedicated body builder. With hard training, the maximum amount of muscle that can be built in a year will be less than 8lb (3.6kg). That represents a gain of two and a half ounces (71g) each week, or a third of an ounce (9.5g) a day. And only 22% of muscle is protein. So an increased protein consumption of less than a tenth of an ounce (2.8g) a day — about a quarter of a teaspoonful — is all that is needed to bring about the greatest possible muscle gain assuming 100% conversion. Yet body builders often think

that the more steaks you can eat, the more muscle you will be able to build!

What can influence your ability to make more muscle are either a poor digestion of protein or a deficiency of the vitamins that convert amino acids into muscle. Poor digestion of protein, although rare, is usually the result of diminished secretion of hydrochloric acid in the stomach. Hydrochloric acid is made by the action of a zinc dependent enzyme, carbonic anhydrase. So adequate zinc is an important factor. However, the nutrient that does more for the metabolism than any other is vitamin B_6. It is involved in protein digesting enzymes, absorption mechanisms for amino acids, converting amino acids into other amino acids and breaking down amino acids to use for energy.

Amino acids and growth hormones

Much attention has recently been directed towards the amino acids l-ornithine and l-arginine. This is because a hormone produced in the pituitary gland, called somatotrophin, or growth hormone, may be influenced by these amino acids. Somatotrophin stimulates muscle formation in the developing years of childhood, after which levels decline. This hormone requires the amio acid ornithine, derived from arginine, to be produced. Arginine itself is also needed in protein synthesis. Some preliminary evidence suggests that supplementing these may stimulate muscle production, however a number of studies have shown inconclusive results using these amino acids. One of the theoretical dangers of supplementing large amounts of arginine is for those carrying or exposed to the herpes virus. This virus lives off arginine and hence may be activated by supplementing arginine.

Nutrients and sports injuries

Usually as a result of over-training or too rapid increases in exercise among less fit people, sports injuries are frequent. These include torn or inflamed muscles, ligaments and tendons, either affecting the muscle itself or its point of attachment on bone. More serious are problems affecting cartilage within joints, such as knee joints. The parts of the body likely to be affected depend on the sport. Runners frequently develop knee problems, while tennis players often develop shoulder problems. Although nutrition is not involved in the injury itself vitamins C, E and zinc help to effect repair to damaged tissue.

Joint problems are also more likely to develop in those who are low in calcium and possibly manganese. One of the first signs of manganese deficiency in animals is knee problems. Muscle stiffness can also occur in an aerobic exercise (for example a sprint) when the exercise is so demanding that not enough oxygen can be provided from respiration. This can can occur in so-called aerobic exercise when the participant is using undeveloped muscle groups. It occurs because glucose gets metabolized into lactic acid when insufficient oxygen is present and this builds up in muscles causing temporary stiffness.

PART SIX

WORKING OUT YOUR OPTIMUM NUTRITION

CHAPTER 6.1

Working out your ideal diet

—OVERVIEW—

What is the optimum diet? Obviously there is no one super diet that is perfect for everyone. We all have different preferences for taste and our individual differences means that our needs for certain nutrients can vary enormously. However there are several essential nutrients and underlying nutritional principles that hold for us all. Any diet can therefore be judged and worked out by these criteria. Below is a list of twelve aspects of diet to consider when working out your ideal diet:

1. Balance between fat, protein and carbohydrates.
2. Acid/Alkaline balance.
3. Choice of vitamin and mineral rich foods.
4. Intake of sugar.
5. Intake of salt.
6. Overall intake of stimulants.
7. Amount of meat vs chicken, fish and vegetable protein.
8. Intake of fibre.
9. Intake of water.
10. Intake of additives, preservatives and anti-nutrients.
11. Intake of essential fatty acids.
12. Amount of raw food and the frequency of frying.

However, nutrition isn't just about working out the idea diet, but also helping people to apply these principles in real life. As well as helping you work out your own ideal diet, this chapter also provides useful tips to help you change your diet for the better.

Throughout this book you will have been introduced to the many different qualities that make up a good diet. The purpose of this chapter is to help you decide what is your ideal diet and to put such a diet into practice.

Any dietary habits are not static, in the sense that both preferences change and the process of improving diet takes time. For example, if you have a sweet tooth or like salty foods it takes some time on a low salt or sugar diet, before the craving for these foods is no longer there. Many people then find that not only do they not crave the foods they used to, but very salty or sweet foods are actually distasteful.

Long-term goals

Therefore it is better to set realistic dietary changes, rather than ideal targets, in the knowledge that you will reach your ideals in time. The practical work following asks you to identify your ideal long-term goals for your diet. These may be things which you don't yet feel able to achieve, but would like to in the long term.

Make a list of all your long-term goals for your diet.

For example 'I don't eat foods with additives.'

'I don't eat foods with added sugar.'

'I eat, on average, four pieces of fruit a day.'

Make your statements as positive and concise as possible. Avoid words like 'should' or 'try' or vague statements like 'I'll try to cut down on . . .'

1. ....

2. ....

3. ....

4. ....

5. ....

6. ....

7. ....

8. ....

9. ....

10. ....

Of course, many of these rules you may wish to qualify. For example, while you may wish to avoid sugar totally when preparing your own food, you may wish to relax these goals on infrequent occasions when eating out, or when being entertained by friends. It is still good to become aware of your long-term intentions.

Short-term targets

Using the following table, build yourself your optimum diet for the next month only. The table includes a list of eleven key dietary principles to follow as closely as possible. It then contains two columns of foods and food categories. Those on the left are generally good for you. Those on the right are generally bad for you. However, there are many exceptions. For example, if you are allergic to milk products then yogurt, listed on the left, will not be good for you, nor will milk or other milk products. If you are not allergic to milk, then there is no reason to avoid milk or milk products completely.

The foods on the left are generally high in specific nutrients, while the foods on the right generally contain an anti-nutrient, stimulant, carcinogen or common allergen. See if you can work out what's special about these foods.

Your optimum diet

The basic principles behind this diet:

1. Make sure at least half your diet consists of ALKALINE forming foods which are all vegetables, fruits, sprouted seeds, yogurt, almonds, brazils, buckwheat.
2. The rest of your diet consists of ACID forming foods such as grains, pulses, nuts, seeds, eggs, cheese, fish and poultry.
3. Eat all food as raw as possible. All cooking destroys some vitamins and breaks down the fibre in food.
4. When using oils other than for cooking (salad dressings, spreads, mayonnaise) use cold pressed sunflower, sesame or safflower oils.
5. Drink at least half a pint of water a day, between meals. For other drinks try diluted fruit juices and herb teas.
6. Avoid foods with added salt. Don't add salt to your cooking or your food. It isn't needed.
7. Avoid sugar and other foods with concentrated sweetness. Honey and maple syrup are marginally better. Dilute fruit juice and soak dried fruit.
8. Avoid fatty meats like beef, pork and lamb, and other high fat foods. Have more vegetarian sources of protein.
9. Avoid 'processed' and 'fast' foods with long lists of preservatives and additives.
10. Avoid frying foods. Grill or bake instead. If you do fry use olive oil or a small amount of butter for as short a time as possible.
11. Avoid regular consumption of tea or coffee. On average, don't drink more than a glass of wine, spirit or pint of beer a day.

Increase these	Avoid these	Decrease these
☐ Beetroot and carrots	☐ Sugar and honey	☐
☐ Wheatgerm and whole grains	☐ Salt and salted foods	☐
☐ Citrus fruit and green peppers	☐ Preservatives and additives	☐
☐ Eggs (not fried)	☐ Chocolate	☐
☐ Dandelion coffee	☐ Coffee	☐
☐ Herb teas	☐ Tea	☐
☐ Bananas and apples	☐ Cigarettes	☐
☐ Seaweed (nori)	☐ Tap water	☐
☐ Tropical fruits	☐ Alcohol	☐
☐ Almonds and brazils	☐ Milk	☐
☐ Yogurt	☐ All milk products	☐
☐ Fish and chicken (free-range)	☐ Beef, pork and lamb	☐
☐ Sesame and sunflower seeds	☐ Parsley, parsnips, celery	☐
☐ Nuts, lentils and beans	☐ Yeast containing foods	☐
☐ Onions and garlic	☐ Soya containing foods	☐
☐ Spring water and fruit juice	☐ Wheat products	☐
	☐ Added wheat bran	☐

Notes

....

....

....

....

....

....

....

....

Turning your attention back to your long-term goals, pick one goal and ask yourself 'What would be an achievable target just for the next month?' For example, if you're a chocolate addict you may feel that you could avoid chocolate completely for one month. However, you cannot imagine being able to avoid coffee altogether. In this example you would set yourself a realistic target for coffee for one month, and tick chocolate in the 'AVOID THESE' column, and coffee in the 'DECREASE THESE' column, perhaps writing 'maximum two cups a day'.

Go through each long-term goal, working out an achievable short-term target. There is a space for notes where you may write other short-term targets, for example 'Eat four pieces of fruit a day'. On the left hand side tick any foods that are good for you and you wish to eat more of (even if you're already eating them). There's nothing wrong with ticking every box.

Just in case you've been over-optimistic, here's a simple test. Pick out the three hardest targets you've set and ask yourself honestly what per cent chance you give yourself of completing these. For example, if you think you have a 50% chance of completing one target then the target is too hard. It is better to succeed in changing your diet gradually, than to shoot for the moon and then give up and go back to your old habits because you couldn't meet your own aspirations.

Tips for reducing or avoiding . . .

Sugar comes in many forms. It's in fruit and complex carbohydrates, as well as chocolate and drinks (when we add it). Don't think of all sugar as bad. However, if you've become 'hooked' on sweet foods with added sugar, then that's what needs to be changed. But its no good avoiding refined sugar if you just add honey or maple syrup instead, or take up eating handfuls of dried fruit. Only by gradually decreasing the overall sweetness of your food will you become used to, and prefer, a less sweet taste. Limit or avoid added sugar in hot drinks. Even better, switch to herb teas or coffee substitutes, many of which are slightly sweet anyway. Use fruit instead of cereal. Have starters instead of puddings. When you crave something sweet eat fresh fruit instead. Dilute fruit juice and soak dried fruit. All these reduce the overall sweetness of foods and drinks.

Salt brings out the flavour in foods. So when coming off salt use more herbs or vegetable stock (try Vecon) to add flavour. If you are not the cook start by not adding salt, even though some may have been used in cooking. Then ask that food is cooked without salt. After all, other people can always add theirs afterwards. Once you have become essentially salt free, the small amount you'll get, for example when eating out, will not harm you.

Chocolate almost always contains sugar too. So which are you addicted to? If you think it's chocolate you can always wean yourself off by eating non-chocolate (and healthier) sweets like Kalibu bars and Take-Off bars, made with carob, or Jordan's Crunchy bars or Shepherdboy Sunflower bars, all available from any health food shop. If you think you're addicted to both and would find total avoidance hard, allow yourself to eat the infrequent Take-Off bar or Sunflower bar when desperate. Both of these are sugar and chocolate free, although they're still quite sweet.

Tea can be drunk in many strengths. Even four tea leaves strongly flavours water. So start by making weaker tea, and using a smaller cup. Luaka, an excellent Ceylon tea, is low in tannin and caffeine.

Coffee contains three stimulants: caffeine, theobromine and theophylline. So decaffeinated coffee is only a bit better for you. Coffee is also extremely addictive. It is often best to go all out and avoid it completely. You may feel rough for up to four days but most people then find the craving is much less and often experience better energy. There are good coffee alternatives from chicory to dandelion coffees and grain coffees. Try them all. They're all different and you are bound to like one.

Alcohol often starts out as a social habit. How best to reduce alcohol may depend on your social life. Many people believe that it would be no fun to be with a group of friends and be sober when they're a little drunk. In fact, research has shown that people feel drunk, when given alcohol free lagers surreptitiously. In the same way, non-drinkers often report feeling good at parties with people who are more relaxed and less inhibited as a result of some alcohol. So you don't actually miss out on a good time. You may find it easier to decide not to drink at lunchtime, or not to drink during the week, or to limit what you drink, or the amount you drink. When you drink less, treat yourself when you do drink by having champagne or a good bottle of wine. After all, you will have saved yourself money by drinking less and good wines tend to be better for you.

Red meat includes beef, pork, lamb and game. There are two factors to consider. One is the fat content and the other is the use of antibiotics and hormones in feed. Lamb tends to be lower in antibiotics and hormones, while game is lower in both. Many people find it easiest to start by avoiding beef and pork, while eating lamb or game once or twice a week. They then progress to eating only fish and chicken, only fish, or no meat or fish at all. Total avoidance of all meat and fish is not necessarily healthier and is a personal decision. Some people wean themselves off meat and fish by allowing themselves meat or fish once a month. Most experience a diminished liking for these foods once decreased.

Milk is only advisable to avoid if an allergy is known or suspected. Good alternatives are soya milk, or nut cream, made by blending nuts and water (cashews are particularly good). Also drink herb teas that don't require milk.

Wheat is only advisable to avoid completely if an allergy is known or suspected. However, it is good not to have a diet dependent on bread. Alternatives are oat cakes, rice cakes, rye bread, pumpernickel bread, rye crispbread and home-made corn bread. Sauces can be thickened with maize flour (wholemeal corn flour) and pastries made with corn and almond meal. There are many oat-based cereals.

To help you get started here are some 'Vitality Recipes' giving simple suggestions for breakfast, lunch and dinner, including easy packed lunches and alternative drinks and snacks.

Eating for vitality

Drinks and snacks

Instead of tea, try herb teas (Celestial Seasonings make some irresistible ones), or Rooibosch tea (with milk, if you like). For real tea addicts, Luaka tea is lowest in tannin and caffeine.

Instead of coffee, try dandelion coffee (Symington's or Dandex) or Barleycup. Decaffeinated coffee is a second best — it still contains two other stimulants.

Drink at least half a pint of spring water a day — it tastes good, especially with ice and lemon.

Fruit juice is good — but check the label for added sugar. Dilute with spring water.

One of the drinks above, with fresh fruit or dried fruit, and perhaps some cashews or pecan nuts, make an ideal snack.

Five breakfast ideas

Natural unsweetened yogurt with any of these: fresh fruit, dried fruit, wheatgerm, desiccated coconut, sunflower seeds, ground sesame seeds, cashews, hazelnuts, almonds (whole or ground).

Muesli (check the label for sugar — or make your own) moistened with yogurt, skimmed milk, soya milk or fruit juice (apple is good). Add extra fruit, nuts or seeds.

Eggs (boiled or poached — not fried) with wholewheat toast or whole rye crispbread or oatcakes or rice cakes (available from health food shops).

Fruit cocktail: liquidize 3 tbs desiccated coconut and ½ tsp vanilla essence with some ice and 8oz (250g) fruit. Try banana and grated apple, orange and banana, orange and peach/nectarine, or a mix of strawberries, raspberries, red and black currants.

Fruit milkshake: chop 4oz fresh fruit (see suggestions above) and blend with 2 tbs ground almonds, 2 tbs desiccated coconut and some ice. Add ½ pt skim or soya milk and liquidize again. Add honey or maple syrup if you like (taste it first!).

Easy packed lunches

All these can be taken to work in a plastic container.

Coleslaw: Finely chop 8 oz (225g) white or red cabbage, 4 oz (125g) carrots, 2 oz (50g) onion. Add 2 oz (50g) walnuts, 2 oz (50g) raisins and just enough (salt and sugar free) mayonnaise to cover. Eat with some celery, carrot sticks, almonds and follow with fresh fruit.

Potato salad: Dice 1 lb (450g) cold boiled potatoes. Add 4 blades fresh chives (or dried) and enough mayonnaise to coat. Add a hardboiled egg or 1 oz (25g) grated cheese for a more substantial meal. Follow with fresh fruit.

Baked potato: Buy one at a takeaway shop (without butter) and add a home-made filling of cottage cheese, chives and cucumber. Follow with fresh fruit or dried fruit and nuts.

Avocado dip: Mash one ripe avocado and add 2 tablespoons natural yogurt, freshly ground pepper and some Vegit (available from health food shops). Eat with pieces of carrot, celery, cucumber, red or green pepper, green beans, radish, cauliflower or spring onions.

Five starters and desserts

Vegetable soup: Fry one large chopped onion, and 2 lb chopped mixed vegetables, then dissolve a salt-free vegetable stock cube in boiling water, add herbs to taste and pour on to vegetables. Simmer for 30 minutes.

Californian Gold: Slice fresh fruit (try apple, banana, nectarine, kiwi fruit and grapes) and serve with hazelnuts, cottage cheese and bean or alfalfa sprouts. With vegetable soup, this can make a complete meal.

Humus: Soak chick peas overnight, boil until tender (about 45 minutes) and blend to a paté consistency with olive oil, garlic, parsley, cumin, pepper, plenty of lemon juice and tahini (sesame spread) and a little cottage cheese. Serve with wholemeal bread or oatcakes.

Fruit fool: Stew 8 oz (225g) dried apricots and liquidize with ¼ tsp natural vanilla essence, 8 lf oz (225g) natural yogurt, and 8 oz (225g) curd cheese. Whisk 2 egg whites and fold into the mixture. Leave in the fridge until needed.

Tea-time treats: Cut 4 oz (125g) softened butter into 6 oz (175g) wholemeal flour with a knife until texture is crumb-like. Bind with water, roll out and use to line tartlet tins. Fill each with a teaspoon of walnuts and a teaspoon of honey and bake until brown at 350°F (175°C) or gas mark 4. Only as a special treat please!

Five main meals

Fish pie: Steam 10 oz (250g) white fish and 10 oz colouring-free smoked haddock for 15 minutes. Meanwhile, make a bechamel sauce with 1 oz (25g) butter, 1 tbs wholemeal flour and ½ pt skim milk.

Mix together fish and sauce with 8 oz (225g) prawns, 4 oz (125g) freshly sliced mushrooms, 2 tsp mixed herbs and freshly ground pepper. Place in oven-proof dish and top with 2 lb (900g) potatoes mashed with milk and pepper. Sprinkle with 4 oz (125g) grated cheese and bake for 30 minutes at 400°F (200°C) or gas mark 6. Serve with fresh peas or beans or a salad.

Stuffed marrow: Bring 2½ cups water to the boil, add 1 cup brown rice and simmer for 45 minutes. Meanwhile 'sauté' 1 chopped medium-size onion in ¼ inch water in a frying pan until just soft. Add 4 oz (125g) chopped mushrooms, 8 oz (225g) chopped tomatoes, 2 tsp mixed herbs and a low salt vegetable stock cube, and cook for 2 minutes.

Cut a medium-size marrow in half lengthways and scoop out the seeds and soft pulp. Add the rice to the vegetable mixture together with 6 oz (150g) chopped hazelnuts or almonds. Pile into the marrow halves and bake (in a roasting bag) for 30 minutes at 400°F (200°C), or until marrow is soft.

Remove from bag, sprinkle with 6 oz (150g) grated cheese. Serve with a mixed salad which includes avocado and hazelnuts.

Millet burgers: mix together 1 finely chopped large onion, 3 oz (75g) grated cheddar, 6 oz (150g) cooked millet flakes or grain, ¼ tsp mustard powder, pepper, 1 tsp thyme, 1 tsp marjoram, 1 egg and some butter.

Form into burger shapes, dot with a little olive oil and put under medium hot grill for 10 minutes each side.

Serve with Waldorf salad — celery, apples, walnuts and mayonnaise mixed half-and-half with yogurt.

Spaghetti: Chop and fry 1 large onion and 3 cloves of garlic in olive oil. Add 1 lb mushrooms, 1 lb tomatoes, 1½ oz tomato purée, herbs and a salt free vegetable stock cube dissolved in water.

Simmer for 20 minutes. Pour over buckwheat spaghetti and serve with green salad — watercress, chicory, iceberg lettuce or endive, cucumber, green pepper, alfalfa sprouts, in an oil and vinegar dressing with herbs (fresh if possible).

Chick pea feast: Soak overnight and boil (for 45 minutes) 6 oz (150g) chick peas. Mix with 3 roughly chopped hardboiled eggs, 7 oz (200g) flaked tuna and 1 small finely chopped onion.

Into a screwtop jar put 1 tbs vinegar, 2 tbs cold-pressed vegetable oil, 3 tbs chopped parsley, 1 tbs chopped chives, ½ tsp mustard powder and some freshly milled black pepper. Pour over the chick pea mix and serve with tomato salad — sliced tomatoes and onion rings with marjoram, olive oil and lemon juice.

Working out your ideal supplement programme

Most people can benefit from nutritional supplements. But, in case you wondered, you don't have to take thirty different supplements every day! Most people's needs can be compressed into four or five different supplements. The most common combinations are a Multivitamin (containing A, D, E, C and the B vitamins) a B-complex (which should contain $B_1, B_2, B_3, B_5, B_6, B_{12}$, folic acid, biotin, PABA, choline and inositol) and a multi mineral for all the minerals. Vitamin C is usually taken separately since the basic optimum requirement of 1,000mg (1 gram) makes quite a large tablet without adding in any more nutrients.

Choosing the right supplements

When choosing the right supplements the quantity of each nutrient in the tablet, the quality and the price all need to be taken into account. To be able to judge a supplement by these criteria it is necessary to understand what's written on the label. Depending on the ingredients different laws apply and since these change from time to time, many manufacturers are as confused as members of the public!

The active ingredients

For some products the ingredients have to be listed in weight order, starting with the largest ingredient. This is often confusing since the non-nutrient additives needed to make the tablet are included in this list. For instance, calcium phosphate, which is a 'filler', is often the first ingredient. In this case it does also provide nutritional benefit, so it is a good filler substance to use. Often the chemical name of the nutrient is used (e.g. ergocalciferol for vitamin D) instead of the common vitamin code. Since most supplements are classified as foods the percentage of the RDA per serving must be listed, as well as the amount per tablet. This law was introduced so that when you eat 100g of a cereal, for example, you known how many vitamins you're getting.

Fillers and binders

Not all products have to declare the other ingredients used to make the supplement. These are included for manufacturing reasons. Tablets start off as powders. To get the bulk right 'fillers' are added. 'Binders' are added to give the mixture the right consistency and lubricants are also used. Only when this is done can the mixture be granulated. This turns the powder into small, uneven granules. The granulated mixture is then pressed into tablets under considerable force. Granulating allows the mixture to lock together forming a solid mass. This is often coated with a 'protein coating' to protect the tablet from deterioration which also makes it easier to swallow.

Unfortunately, many tablets also have colouring and flavouring added, as well as a sugar coating. For instance, many vitamin C tablets look orange and taste sweet, since we associate vitamin C with oranges! Vitamin C is almost white and certainly isn't sweet. Nor should your supplement be. As a rule of thumb, only buy supplements that declare their fillers and binders (these are sometimes called excipients), as companies with integrity are usually only too happy to display this information. The following fillers and binders are fine to use and some add extra nutritious properties to the tablet.

> *Dicalcium phosphate* — a natural filler providing calcium and phosphate
> *Cellulose* — a natural binder consisting of plant fibre
> *Alginic acid/sodium alginate* — a natural binder from seaweed
> *Gum acacia/gum arabic* — a natural vegetable gum
> *Calcium or magnesium stearate* — a natural lubricant
> *Silica* — a natural lubricant
> *Zein or protein coating* — a corn protein for coating the tablet
> *Brazil wax* — a natural coating from palm trees.

Chart 6.2.1 — *Natural fillers, binders, lubricants and coatings*

'Free from sugar, starch and gluten . . .'

Many better tablets will declare that the product is free from sugar and gluten. If you are milk or yeast allergic do check that it is also free from lactose (milk sugar) and yeast. Some B vitamins are derived from yeast so you need to be careful. If in doubt, call the company and ask for an independent assay of the ingredients. The better companies will supply this information. Sometimes, glucose (dextrose) or fructose is used to sweeten a tablet and yet the tablet still declares 'no sugar'. These are best avoided. A small amount of fructose is the least evil if you're having difficulty enticing a child to take vitamins. Any other preservatives or flavouring agents should be avoided unless they are natural. For instance, pineapple essence is a natural additive.

Capsules *vs* Tablets

Capsules are made of gelatin, which is an animal product, and is therefore not suitable for vegetarians. Some capsules also contain the preservative called methyl paraben, which stops the gelatin decaying or dissolving. In some countries, such as the UK, this is banned although the law is rarely enforced. Most vitamins can be provided as tablets. For instance natural vitamin E comes in two forms: d-alpha tocopheryl acetate (oil) or d-alpha tocopherol succinate (powder). Both are equally potent iu for iu though not weight for weight.

Natural *vs* synthetic

A lot of rubbish has been said about the pros of natural vitamins. First of all, many products claiming to be natural simply aren't. By law, a certain percentage of a product must be natural for the product to be declared 'natural'. The percentage varies from country to country. By careful wording some supplements sound natural but really aren't. For instance, 'vitamin C with rosehips' invariably means synthetic vitamin C with added rosehips, although it is often confused to mean vitamin C from rosehips. So which is better?

By definition, a synthetic vitamin must contain all the properties of the vitamin found in nature. If it doesn't then the chemists haven't done their job properly. This is the case for vitamin E. Natural d-alpha tocopherol succinate is 36% more potent than the synthetic vitamin E called dl-alpha tocopherol. (In this case the 'l' dictates the chemical difference.) So natural vitamin E, usually derived from wheat germ or soya oil, is better weight for weight that synthetic.

However, synthetic vitamin C (ascorbic acid) has the same biological potency as the natural, according to Dr Linus Pauling.[42] Indeed, most vitamin C is synthesized by taking a 'natural' sugar such as dextrose, and two chemical reactions later you have ascorbic acid. This is little different from the chemical reactions that take place in animals who convert sugar to vitamin C. Vitamin C derived from, say, acerola berries, which is the most concentrated source, is also considerably bulkier and more expensive. A 1,000mg tablet would be five times as large as a normal tablet (since acerola is 20% vitamin

C) and would cost you ten times as much!

However, vitamins derived from natural sources may contain an unknown element that increases their potency. For instance, with vitamin E this may well be octacosanol, a nutritional substance found in vegetable oils. Vitamin C is found in nature together with the bioflavonoids. These are active nutrients that appear to increase the potency of vitamin C, particularly in its capacity of strengthening the capillaries, which are tiny blood vessels. The best source of bioflavonoids is citrus fruit so the addition of citrus bioflavonoids to vitamin C tablets is a step closer to nature.

Watch out for elemental minerals

Minerals in mutivitamin and mineral tablets often omit the 'elemental' value of the compound, stating only the amount of the mineral compound. For instance, zinc gluconate or zinc orotate 100mg, will provide only 10mg of zinc and 90mg of orotic acid, which is misleadingly called B_{13} since it is not a B vitamin. Since it's the mineral you're after check the figures carefully. If your supplement says 'Zinc Gluconate (providing 5mg zinc) 50mg' you're getting 5mg of zinc. Otherwise, you may have to call the manufacturer. Most good companies declare this information either on the label or in product literature.

When a mineral is attached to a compound such as an amino acid this is called 'chelated' from the Greek work meaning a claw. Chelated minerals are often absorbed twice as well, and, in a sense mimic what the body does normally. When we ingest a mineral it must be combined with an amino acid, which is a constituent of protein, to be absorbed. So minerals normally have to compete for amino acids — and not all win. Zinc, for instance, has to compete with lead for the same chelating agents. By providing already chelated minerals absorption is far better.

What about sustained release?

Some vitamins are called prolonged, sustained or time-released implying that the ingredients are not all made available for absorption in one go. This can be useful when taking large amounts of water soluble vitamins such as B complex or vitamin C. However, this depends on the person and the dosage. For example, many people are able to absorb and use 1,000mg of vitamin C taken in one dose. Taking this in sustained release form would be little benefit. However, if you take three 1,000mg tablets each day, sustained release would allow you to take them all in one go. Since sustained release vitamins are more expensive one has to weigh up the pros and cons. Sustained release products should be taken with food or they may pass through the body too quickly and before releasing their nutrients.

There is no point in having a sustained release fat soluble vitamin such as vitamin A, D or E as these store in the body.

Which supplements are good value?

For a supplement to be good value it must be well made, well formulated and well priced. The quality of manufacture is hard to assess unless you have an advanced chemistry laboratory in your back room! However, there are three simple tests you can do:

Testing the quality

1. Are there the stated number of tablets in the bottle? (We tested one company and found an average of 95 tablets instead of 100!)
2. Is the tablet coated all round and therefore easy to swallow? (Uncoated or badly coated tablets can break up or taste bad.)
3. Does the label tell you everything you need to know? (The better the company the more information they will want to give you.)

The ideal formulas

Every nutritionist has different ideas about the 'best' blend of vitamins and minerals in supplements, which is reflected in the ever-growing range to choose from. The ideal formulation ultimately depends on your needs, however there are certain basic formulations which act as the building blocks for your Personal Health Programme. These are a multivitamin, a B complex, a vitamin C, and a multimineral tablet. These recommended formulas will cover the basic nutrient requirements for optimum health. Depending on your signs of deficiency you may also need to add extra B vitamins or individual minerals.

B complex — This should contain at least 25mg of B_1, B_2, PABA, choline and inositol, and 50mg of B_3, B_5 and B_6, as well as 10mcg B_{12}, 50mcg folic acid and 50mcg biotin.

Multivitamin — This should contain 7,500iu of A, 400iu of D, 100iu of E, 250mg of C and 25mg of B_1, B_2, B_3, B_5 and B_6. (If it is to be taken on its own as a complete multivitamin and mineral extra B_{12}, folic acid, biotin, PABA, choline, inositol and minerals are needed, as well as more vitamin C.) Often calcium, magnesium, iron, zinc and manganese are included as these are frequently deficient.

Multimineral — This should provide 150mg calcium, 75mg magnesium, 10mg iron, 10mg zinc, 2.5mg manganese, 20mcg chromium, 25mcg selenium. (Selenium is often excluded as it is better absorbed on an empty stomach.)

Vitamin C — This should provide 1,000mg of vitamin C *with* at least 25mg of bioflavonoids.

When should you take vitamin supplements?

Now that you've worked out what to take you'll want to know when to take them. This depends not only on what is technically best, but also on your lifestyle. If taking supplements twice a day would mean that you'd forget the second lot, you're probably best advised to take them all at once! After all, nature supplies them all in one go, with a meal. Here are the 'ten commandments' of supplement taking:

THE TEN COMMANDMENTS OF SUPPLEMENT TAKING

1. Take vitamins and minerals 15 minutes before, during or after a meal.
2. Selenium is better absorbed on an empty stomach — try first thing in the morning.
3. Don't take B vitamins late at night if you have difficulty sleeping.
4. Take multiminerals or dolomite tablets in the evening — these help you to sleep.

5. If you're taking two or more B complex's or vitamin C's take one at each meal.
6. If you are anaemic (iron deficient) take extra iron with vitamin C. Avoid 'ferric' forms of iron.
7. If you are zinc deficient take extra zinc with vitamin B_6.
8. If you know you are copper deficient only take this with ten times as much zinc e.g. 0.5mg copper to 5mg zinc.
9. If you are taking glucomannan take most of your vitamin supplements with breakfast and most of your glucomannan with lunch or dinner.
10. Always take your supplements. Irregular supplementation doesn't work.

What improvements in my health can I expect?

Vitamins and minerals are not drugs so you shouldn't expect an overnight improvement in your health. Most people on Personal Health Programmes have experienced definite improvement in health within three months. This is the shortest length of time that you should experiment with a programme. The earliest noticeable health changes are increased energy, more emotional stability, and improvements in the condition of your hair and skin. Your health will continue to improve as long as you are following the right programme. My health is still improving five years later! If you do not experience any noticeable improvement in three months it is best to see a nutrition consultant.

How often should I reassess my needs?

Certainly at the beginning your needs will change and a reassessment every three months is sensible. Your nutrient needs should decrease as you get healthier. Remember, you need optimum nutrition most when you are stressed. So when emergencies occur, or you're working especially hard make sure you eat well and take your supplements every day.

Are there any side-effects?

Vitamins are unlikely to produce serious side-effects. However, you may find that your bowels will be looser if you are taking 1,000 to 3,000mg of vitamin C. Also, your urine will become more yellow as a result of B_2, riboflavine. Vitamin B_3 in the nicotinic acid form (called niacin in the US or Australia) is a vasodilator. This means that your capillaries dilate causing a 'blushing' sensation. This can be quite pronounced, and although good for you, not everybody likes it. So proceed with caution. 100mg of B_3 is enough to cause this effect.

If you do get any unpleasant effects shortly after starting your programme these are more often than not 'withdrawal symptoms' if you've stopped drinking coffee or eating sugar. They'll go away in a week. However, if they don't go away stop the supplements and see what happens. You may be one of the rare people allergic to a filler or binder or yeast, which is used in some supplements. In these situations it is best to see your doctor.

Can vitamins be dangerous?

All food substances are toxic if taken in excess and vitamins and minerals are no exception. However, the fact that vitamins can be toxic has been ridiculously exploited. For instance, a recent article reporting toxicity of vitamin B_6 at levels of 2,000mg to 6,000mg per day, which is at least eight times greater than the *maximum* optimum level suggested, was used as ammunition to ban high dose B_6 supplements. The most toxic vitamins are vitamin A which can cause death at levels of 1 million iu in one dose and D. With the highest supplement of vitamin A containing 7,500iu per tablet, one would have to take 134 tablets in one go! Compared to common pain killers even vitamin A is remarkably untoxic.

However, since toxicity of some vitamins has not been thoroughly researched it is far better to err on the side of caution.

—CONCLUSION—

Well done! Having completed *The Family Nutrition Workbook* you will have learnt much more than the basics of 'optimum' nutrition. If you've applied the principles discussed to your own diet and lifestyle you'll be feeling healthier too. To show you how your own health has and

will improve I recommend you fill in another Nutrition Programme Questionnaire in three months' time. Then compare which symptoms have gone away.

Wishing you good health,

References

The references listed here represent a fraction of those used in writing this workbook. Many journals now publish research in nutrition and health. These include the *British Medical Journal, The Lancet*, the *American Journal of Clinical Nutrition, Nutrition Reviews, Nutrition and Health* and the *Journal of Orthomolecular Psychiatry*. A useful review journal that abstracts papers on nutrition from many leading journals is the *International Clinical Nutrition Review*. Details on this are obtainable from PO Box 344, Carlingford, New South Wales, 2118, Australia.

1. J. Jenkins, *Am. J. Clin. Nutr.*, 34: 362, 1981.
2. C. Kagan, 'Lysine therapy for Herpes Simplex', *Lancet*, 1:37 (1974).
3. J. Yacenda, 'The Herpes Diet', Felmore Ltd. Health Publications Newsletter No. 5.
4. *A Square Meal for Britain?*, 1981, Bateman Catering Organisation.
5. *Proposals for Nutritional Guidelines for Health Education in Britain*, NACNE 1983, Health Education Council.
6. *The Booker Health Report*, 1985.
7. D. Grant, 1986, *Food Combining for Health*, Thorsons.
8. C. Wright, 1986, *The Wright Diet*, Piatkus.
9. A. Schauss, 1981, *Diet, Crime and Delinquency*, Parker House.
10. R. Gray, 1980, *The Colon Health Handbook*, Rockridge Publishing.
11. C. Paterson, 1983, *Lead vs Health*, p. 17-28, edit. Rutter, Russell Jones, Wiley.
12. H. Needleman, 1979, *N. Engl. J. Med.*, 300, 689.
13. *Lead and Health*, 1980, DHSS Working Party Report (HMSO).
14. R. Lansdown and Yule, chapter in *Lead vs Health* (see ref. 11).
15. G. Winneke, chapter in *Lead vs Health* (see ref. 11).
16. C. Pfeiffer, 1978, *J. Ortho. Psych.*, 7:2. and 1982, *Biological Pysch.*, 17:4.
17. American Dental Association Factsheet, 1984.
18. S. Ziff, 1984, *Toxic Time Bomb*, Thorsons.
19. J. Edwardson, 1986, *The Lancet*, February 15 p. 354.
20. B. Weiss, 1980, *Science*, 207:1487-1488 see also B. Weiss, 1980, *Science*, 207, March.
21. P. Dallman, 1981, *Nutrition in the 1980s: Constrains on our knowledge*, p. 87, eds. N. Selvey and P. White, New York: Alan R. Riss.
22. G. Youcha, 1982, 'The Cortisone Dilemma', *Science Digest*, January.
23. Mr. A. McCance and E. M. Widdowson, 1960, *The Composition of Foods*, HMSO.
24. A. Knowles, 1985, Personal communication to author.
25. A. Streissguth, 1979, *New Scientist*.
26. C. Pfeiffer, 1987, *Schizophrenia and Mental Illness: The Nutrition Connection*, Thorsons.
27. Office of Population Censuses and Surveys, 1984 report (available from St Catherine's

House, Kingsway WC2).

28. R. Passwater, 1975, *Supernutrition for a Healthy Heart*, Thorsons, p. 46.

29. Alfin-Slater, 1975, report at International Congress of Nutrition in Kyoto, Japan and in *Los Angeles Times*, October 2.

30. B. Hirshowitz *et al*, 1976, *Brit. J. Plastic Surgery*.

31. P. Herbert, 1977, *Medical World News*, February.

32. *Diet and Coronary Heart Disease*, 1974, Report of the Advisory Panel of the Committee of Medical Aspects of Food Policy on Diet in Relation to Cardiovascular and Cerebrovascular Disease.

33. W. Martin, 1977, *Medical Heroes and Heretics*, Devin Adair.

34. E. Shute *The Heart and Vitamin E*, 1969, The Shute Foundation for Medical Research, London, Canada, see also W. Shute and H. Taub, 1969, *Vitamin E for Ailing and Healthy Hearts*, Pyramid House, New York.
W. Shute, 1978, *The Vitamin E Book*, Keats.

35. R. Passwater, 1976, *Prevention* magazines, January-May, July-September, Rodale Press.

36. E. Ginter, 1973, *Science*, 179:702.
E. Ginter, 1978, *Lipid Research*, 16:167-220.
E. Ginter, 1982, 'Vitamin C in the Control of Hypercholesterolaemia in Man', in *Vitamin C: New Clinical Applications in Immunology, Lipid Metabolism and Cancer*, ed. Hanck, Hans Huber, Bern, p. 137-152.

37. P. Turlapaty *et al*, 1980, *Science*, 208: 198-200 see also M. Speich *et al*, 1980, *Clinical Chemistry*, 26:12:1662-1665.
J. Swales, 1982, *Brit. Med. J.*, 285:1377-1378.

38. R. Cathcart, 1984, *Medical Hypotheses* 14:423-433.

39. S. Davies, chapter in 1984-85 *Yearbook of Nutritional Medicine*, ed. J. Bland, Keats, 1985.

40. M. Golden, 1977, *Lancet* ii: 1057-9.

41. G. Eby *et al*, 1984, *Antimicrobial Agents and Chemotherapy*, 25:1:20-24.

42. L. Pauling, 1986, *How To Live Longer and Feel Better*, Freeman, p. 163-180.

43. L. Pauling, 1986, *How To Live Longer and Feel Better*, Freeman, p. 163-180.

44. G. Schrauzer, 1959, *Bio-organic Chemistry*, 2:4.

45. C. Pfeiffer, 1987, *Schizophrenia and Mental Illness*, Thorsons.

46. NASA report, 1982, American Medical Association symposium, Florida see also M. Korcak, 1982, *J. Am. Med. Assoc.*, 247:8.

47. M. Colgan, 1983, *Your Personal Vitamin Profile*, Blond & Briggs.

48. A. Eyton, 1982, *F-Plan Diet*, Penguin.

49. W. McArdle, 1984, chapter in *Medical Applications of Clinical Nutrition*, ed. J. Bland, Keats.

50. C. Hollenbeck, 1983, *Am. J. Clin. Nutr.*, 38:498, 1983.

51. A. Hoffer, 1980, *Nutrients to Age Without Senility*, Pivot.

52. C. Pfeiffer, 1975, *Mental and Elemental Nutrients*, Keats.

53. R. Mohs *et al.*, 1979, *Am. J. Psych.*, 136:1275.

54. L. Byerley, 1985, *Amer. J. Clin. Nutr.*, 41, 4, 666. See also C. Kunz, 1984, *Int. J. for Vitamin Nutr. Research*, 54, 141.

55. C. Donangelo, 1984, *Nutr. Reports Intern.* 30, 5, 1157. See also M. Ruz, 1984, *Nutr. Research*, 4, 923 and P. Moser, 1983, *Amer. J. Clin. Nutr.*, 38, 101.

56. H. Korpela, 1984, *Int. J. Vitamin and Nutr. Research*, 54, 257.

57. J. Steiner, 1984, *Community Dentistry and Oral Epidemiology*, 12, 6, 386.

58. P. Braidwood, 1987, 'Better babies by design' *The Observer Supplement*, 26 April.

59. A. Streissguth, 1979, *New Scientist*.

60. R. Naeye, 1984, *Obstet. and Gynaecol.*, 64, 5, 601.

61. P. Rantakillio, 1978, *Early Hum. Dev.*, 2:371-83.

62. C. Pfeiffer, 1983, *Inter. J. Env. Studies*, 17, 43-56.

63. P. Ylastalo, 1975, *Ann. Chirurgiae et Gynaecol. Fenniae*, 64, 128-134.

64. E. Lodge Rees, 1983, *Trace Elements in Health*, Butterworth, England.

65. *Booker Health Report*, 1986, Booker Health Foods.

66. D. Bryce-Smith, 1987, *The Zinc Solution*, Century Arrow.

67. P. Holford, 1983, *Testing The Effects of Glucomannan on Weight Loss*, ION.

68. K. Cooper, 1978, *The Aerobics Way*, Corgi Books.

69. J. Mayer, 1956, *Am. J. Clin. Nutr.*, 4:169.

Further reading

The following books are recommended for digging deeper into the subjects covered in this book:

Chapter 3.1 The Macronutrients
The Food Scandal, Geoffrey Cannon and Caroline Walker, Century (1984).

Chapter 3.2 The Vitamins
Vitamin Vitality, Patrick Holford, Collins (1985).

Chapter 3.3 The Minerals
Elemental Health, Patrick Holford, Thorsons (1983).

Chapter 3.4 The Essential Fatty Acids
Evening Primrose Oil, Judy Graham, Thorsons (1984).

Chapter 3.5 Special Diets
Raw Energy, Leslie and Susannah Kenton, Century (1984).
Food Combining for Health, Doris Grant and Jean Joice, Thorsons (1984).

Chapter 3.6 Preparing Healthy Food
The Complete Wholefood Cuisine, Nikki and David Goldbeck, Thorsons (1987).
The Here's Health Wholefood Cookery Course, Janette Marshall and Sarah Bounds, Thorsons (1986).

Chapter 3.7 The Anti-Nutrients
Detoxifying Lead, Patrick Holford, ION (1984).
The New E for Additives, Maurice Hanssen, Thorsons (1987).

Chapter 4.2 Boosting Immune Power
Ageless Ageing, Leslie Kenton, Century/Arrow (1986).
Cancer and Its Nutritional Therapies, Passwater, Keats (1978).

Chapter 4.3 Overcoming Allergies
Allergies: Your Hidden Enemy, Theron G. Randolph M.D., and Ralph W. Moss Ph.D., Thorsons (1984).

Chapter 4.4 Nutrition, the Mind and Behaviour
Mental Illness and Schizophrenia: The Nutrition Connection, Dr Carl C. Pfeiffer, Thorsons (1987).

Chapter 4.7 Nutrition and Weight Problems
The Metabolic Diet, Patrick Holford, Ebury Press (1987).

Chapter 5.2 Nutrition for Babies and Children
The Better Pregnancy Diet, Patrick and Liz Holford, Ebury Press (1987).

Chapter 5.3 Nutrition During Pregnancy
The Better Pregnancy Diet, Patrick and Liz Holford, Ebury Press (1987).

Useful addresses

The Association of Nutrition Consultants can refer you to a nutrition consultant in your area. They publish a directory of qualified nutrition consultants trained at the Institute for Optimum Nutrition. To receive the directory please send £1.00 to ANC, Maryland, Croft Road, Hastings, East Sussex.

Foresight provides information and personal advice on the importance of pre-conceptual care and nutrition. For more details send an SAE to *Foresight*, The Old Vicarage, Church Lane, Witley, Godalming, Surrey GU8 5PN.

The Hyperactive Children's Support Group offer help and advice for the families of hyperactive children. Please send an SAE to HACSG Mayfield House, Yapton Road, Barnham, Bognor Regis, West Sussex PO22 0BJ.

The Institute for Optimum Nutrition offers courses and personal consultations with trained nutritionists, including Patrick Holford. They also publish a quarterly magazine, *Optimum Nutrition*, available to ION members. For more details send an SAE to ION, 5 Jerdan Place, London SW6 1BE (Phone: 01-381 5698).

Index